# AETCOM

## Attitude, EThics and COMmunication
### M A N U A L

Learning Modules for MBBS Professional Year I
Competencies for the
Indian Medical Graduate

As Recommended by Medical Council of India

# AETCOM

## Attitude, EThics and COMmunication

MANUAL

Learning Modules for MBBS Professional Year I
Competencies for the
Indian Medical Graduate

As Recommended by Medical Council of India

*Editor*

## Nitin Ashok John

MBBS MD FRSB (London, UK), FASSOPI (India), FAcad Med Edu (Cardiff, UK 2021), FRSPH (London, UK 2021)
GDMLE (Medical Law and Ethics, NLSIU Bengaluru), DIH, PGDHA (Hospital Administration)
MA (Public Administration), European Lifestyle Medicine Organization Certified Graduate

Professor and Head
Department of Physiology
All India Institute of Medical Sciences
Bibinagar, Hyderabad

*Contributors*

### K Rajgopal Shenoy
MBBS MS FRCS (Glasgow)
Professor
Department of Surgery
Ex-Associate Dean—Academics
Kasturba Medical College, and
Consultant Surgeon, Kasturba Hospital
Manipal 576104, Karnataka, India
Manipal Academy of Higher Education (MAHE)

### Sanjay Andrew Rajaratnam
MBBS MD
Professor and Head
Department of Physiology
Coordinator of the Medical Education
Unit Chettinad Hospital and Research Institute
Kelambakkam—Kanchipuram District
Chennai—South India

### Krishna Garg
MBBS MD PhD FIMSA FIAMS FAMS FASI
Ex-Professor and Head
Department of Anatomy
Lady Hardinge Medical College
New Delhi

### Maria Pauline
MBBS MD
Associate Professor
St Johns Medical College
Bangalore

## CBS Publishers & Distributors Pvt Ltd

New Delhi • Bengaluru • Chennai • Kochi • Kolkata • Lucknow • Mumbai
Gujarat • Hyderabad • Jharkhand • Nagpur • Patna • Pune • Uttarakhand

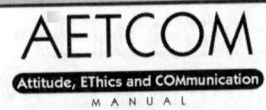

**Attitude, EThics and COMmunication**

M A N U A L

Learning Modules for MBBS Professional Year I
Competencies for the
Indian Medical Graduate
As Recommended by Medical Council of India

**ISBN:** 978-93-89565-78-2

**First Edition: 2020**
   **Reprint:** 2021, 2022, 2024, **2026**

Published by **Satish Kumar Jain** and produced by **Varun Jain** for

## CBS Publishers & Distributors Pvt Ltd

4819/XI Prahlad Street, 24 Ansari Road, Daryaganj, New Delhi 110 002, India
Ph: 011-23289259, 23266838
           Website: www.cbspd.com
           e-mail: delhi@cbspd.com

*Corporate Office:* 204 FIE, Industrial Area, Patparganj, Delhi 110 092
Ph: 011-4934 4934     Fax: 011-4934 4935     e-mail: publishing@cbspd.com; publicity@cbspd.com

### Branches

- **Bengaluru:** Seema House 2975, 17th Cross, K.R. Road, Banasankari 2nd Stage, Bengaluru 560 070 Karnataka, India
  Ph: +91-80-26771678/79     Fax: +91-80-26771680     e-mail: bangalore@cbspd.com
- **Chennai:** 18/8B, Subbarayan Street, Shenoy Nagar, Chennai 600 030, Tamil Nadu, India
  Ph: +91-44-42032115, 45022115     e-mail: chennai@cbspd.com
- **Kochi:** 42/1325, 1326, Power House Road, opposite KSEB, Power House, Ernakulam 682 018 Kochi, Kerala, India
  Ph: +91-484-4059061–65     e-mail: kochi@cbspd.com
- **Kolkata:** 147, Hind Ceramics Compound, 1st Floor, Nilgunj Road, Belghoria, Kolkata 700 056 West Bengal, India
  Ph: +91-33-25633055–56     e-mail: kolkata@cbspd.com
- **Lucknow:** Basement, Khushnuma Complex, 7-Meerabai Marg (behind Jawahar Bhawan) Lucknow 226 001, UP, India
  Ph: +91-522-4000032     e-mail: tiwari.lucknow@cbspd.com
- **Mumbai:** PWD Shed. Gala No. 25/26, Ramchandra Bhatt Marg, Next to JJ Hospital Gate No. 2 Opposite Union Bank of India Noorbaug, Mumbai 400 009, Maharashtra, India
  Ph: +91-22-66661880/89     e-mail: mumbai@cbspd.com

### Representatives

- **Gujarat** • **Hyderabad** • **Jharkhand** • **Nagpur** • **Patna** • **Pune** • **Uttarakhand**

For trade terms please contact customercare@cbspd.com

For general enquiries please contact info@cbspd.com

Printed at: SRK Graphics, Delhi, India

# Preface

It gives us immense pleasure to author the theoretical aspects of *AETCOM: Attitude, EThics and COMmunication Manual— Learning Modules for MBBS Professional Year 1*. The medical students need to be trained, nurtured and groomed in environment of high academic standard with complete awareness regarding the professional qualities and role of physician and need for ethics in medical practice, as students of today will be the practicing doctors of tomorrow.

The present module shall be immensely helpful to gain sufficient knowledge and skills required to understand and practice the intricracies and understand the needs of noble attitude, ethics and communication in medical profession.

The students should understand that the medical profession is a lifelong commitment for learning and gaining knowledge and skills, so as they mature as experts, they should develop the sense of sincerity, originality and noble, humble and sacrificial humane personality. Last but not the least, the doctors should understand the apathy of patient in sickness and their word of solace in empathetic manner goes in long way in developing confidence in patient and facilitate their early recovery.

The lucid, integrated and comprehensive training will be instrumental in developing a confidant doctor. We wish the students all success, seeking honour, becoming reckon, acquiring all prosperity with due humility.

**Nitin Ashok John**
**K Rajgopal Shenoy**
**Sanjay Andrew Rajaratnam**
**Krishna Garg**
**Maria Pauline**

# Contents

# Index of Competencies

Competency based Undergraduate Curriculum for the
Indian Medical Graduate

# What does it Mean to be a Doctor?

*Nitin Ashok John*

## Competencies Addressed

*The student should be able to:*

1. Enumerate and describe professional qualities and roles of a physician
2. Describe and discuss the commitment to lifelong learning as an important part of physician growth
3. Describe and discuss the role of a physician in healthcare system
4. Identify and discuss physician's role and responsibility to society and the community that she/he serves

## ▌ Learning Objective Background

The main aim of introducing this topic is to make students aware of the profession they have chosen as their career, their duties and responsibilities towards the profession and community, prospective challenges they will be exposed to during learning and clinical practices and their career prospects. The students are to be trained and their thinking modulated to achieve excellence in their career and as they proceed in their journey of medical studies, they should be optimistic and charged up with enthusiasm to learn and adapt the clinical acumen and skill so as to achieve the best performance in all medical professional examinations, postgraduate entrance, postgraduate studies and moreover aiming high to touch the skies.

The gist of the learning will be to understand the need of adequate medical knowledge, skills and clinical acumen and acquiring noble virtues and characteristics of selflessness, caring attitude, generosity, dedication and devotion towards patient to become successful doctors.

## INTRODUCTION

The medical profession is a noble and one of the most sought-after careers worldwide. Many of the students nurture the desire to become a doctor from the time of toddler age. The parental pressure at times may force the student to enter the medical profession. The students take this profession by virtue of their hardwork, sincerity, honesty, and devotion towards the academics throughout the schooling and junior college. As they enter into professional college, they experience an environment of professionalism, very different from school life and while in their studies in the medical institute, they undergo various pressure, such as competitive studies for better performance, peer pressure, psychological anxiety regarding future career prospects, longer span of year of studies and so, also regarding delayed settlement in life as compared to their peers in other profession. In the above process, they gradually accustom themselves learning and acquiring clinical skills and knowledge and so, also understanding the privileges, duties, responsibilities, ethics and obligations towards patient and community in medical profession. This chapter helps in understanding the role, responsibilities and commitment of doctors towards patients and society. It also emphasizes the need of continue medical education and upgradation as an essential part in career development for medical professionals.

## GENERAL MEDICAL PRACTITIONER AND SPECIALIST

*The medical students pursuing MBBS (Bachelor of Medicine and Surgery) degree after graduation and completion of internship usually enter clinical practice and are referred as* medical practitioners, and their duties are centered towards promoting, managing and restoring physical and mental health. The medical doctors who are working as 'general duty medical officers' are referred as 'medical physician' while those specializing in internal medicine are referred as 'medical specialist' or depending on the basis of specialization are called pediatrician, ophthalmologist, surgeon, ENT surgeon, obstetrician, gynecologist, radiologist, etc.

## ATTRIBUTES OF A DOCTOR

As a practicing doctor in private practice or in a government institute, a humanistic doctor respects all individuals (healthy or diseased) and is considerate towards the patients and their relatives, provides promotive, curative and preventive health, employs effective communication skills while interacting with patients, imparts unbiased advice, carefully listens to patients' apathy, and is sympathetic towards patients, seeking informed consent in all decisions related to patient's health and patient's healthcare needs and ensures patient's physical wellness.

## PROFESSIONAL QUALITIES OF A PHYSICIAN

1. **Moral intellect practices with responsibility and accountability:** The doctor with moral intellect practices medicine as per the ethical guidelines laid by the medical council with uttermost sincerity, devotion, dedication, commitment, selfless service, sense of responsibility and readiness for accountability for the positive happening or negative mishaps while he/she is applying medical knowledge and skills in treating patients.

2. **Ethical and legal codes of conduct:** A responsible doctor practices principle of informed consent and confidentiality in true sense in his/her healthcare delivery. He/she has adequate knowledge of medico-legal, societal, ethical and humanitarian principles influencing healthcare. Thus, to conclude he/she is aware and able to manage ethical and professional conflicts and abides by ethical and legal codes of conduct and practices guidelines meticulously.

3. **Personal attributes:** He is kind, compassionate, accommodative, humanistic, honest, a better listener towards his/her patient's misery, and provides peace, solace and confidence to the patient for his/her speedy recovery.

4. **Knowledge and skills:** A good doctor shall use all their wits and knowledge, employing all their clinical acumen and skills in saving patient's health and imparting new life.

5. **Practices pertaining to specialization:** A good doctor limits his/her practice to skills and specialization achieved by him/her and tenable as per medical council, government body and health mission guidelines. Never indulge in any medical practices outside his/her domain. He/she is ready to seek second opinion on request of his/her patients.

6. **Professional conduct:** A good doctor maintains his/her conduct towards his/her patients, his/her professional colleagues and community as per professional conduct of noble and dignified approach as recommended by Code of Ethics recommended by Medical Council of India.

7. **Avoids publicity:** A good doctor is humble and believes in services rather than publicity. He/she does not use services of any media for publicity of his/her clinical practices, e.g.

distribution of pamphlets, advertising through TV channels, radio services, etc.

8. **Relevant referrals:** A good doctor never makes unnecessary referrals for investigations or opinion unless condition warrants need in true sense. He/she can identify need for to refer patient who needs specialized or advanced tertiary care.

9. **Growth of the medical profession:** A good doctor is committed to the growth of the medical profession by his/her selfless services to patient and society.

10. **Adequate knowledge of disease and healthcare delivery:** A good doctor has adequate knowledge of anatomy, physiology and pathology of human body especially its organ system especially pertaining to its cellular and biochemical basis and can differentiate between its clinical, behavioural and social perspective. A good doctor can differentially diagnose and interpret investigative data in order to address patient's problems.

11. **Participation in national and regional healthcare program:** A good doctor has adequate knowledge of national and regional healthcare policies and modes to impart an economically viable and effective patient-oriented healthcare.

12. **Communication skills:** A good doctor is an excellent communicator and elicits history of disease from patient/and or his/her relatives; a history that is complete in all aspects and helps to easily diagnose the disease and this is immensely helpful in patient's management.

13. **Practices with caution and care:** A good doctor maintains accurate, detailed and appropriate records of the patient treated by them in order to facilitate follow-up management and if required in cases of medical litigation and administrative frameworks.

14. **Altruism:** A good doctor shall ensure patients interest over self; especially their wishes in reference to preferred line of management. Any error by omission or commission as part of altruism must be disclosed to patient and medical hospital authorities as a noble practice methodology which otherwise is not usually done.

Thus, a good doctor is one who is successful in disease prevention, health promotion and cure, pain and distress alleviation, and able to impart safe rehabilitation and palliative services.

## SUMMARY: QUALITIES OF A GOOD DOCTOR

- A good doctor is caring and loving, compassionate and kind.
- Comforting, assuring, alleviating patient's misery with conscientious mind.
- Listening, accommodating, comforting, energizing patient with peace and confidence.
- Being humanistic, honest, practicing confidentiality in practices bears fruitful concordance.
- Nurture sense of hope, confidence, recovery, rejuvenation, renewing a revive.
- Using all his/her clinical acumen and skills in saving patient's health imparting new life.
- Imbibe with knowledge, optimism, persuasive nature and intellect philosophy.
- Selflessly serving sick and destitute with all his/her might, potential, ability and generosity.

Thus, a student of today will be the doctor of tomorrow and he/she should maintain the dignity and higher standard of attitude, behaviour and ethical practices as a part of this noble profession.

## COMMITMENT OF LIFELONG LEARNING—AN IMPORTANT PART OF A PHYSICIAN'S GROWTH

### INTRODUCTION

The medical physician has a lifelong commitment towards learning and he/she acquires knowledge and skills over the years as cumulative effect achieving excellence by his/her quest and inner drive to acquire, learn and adapt the advances in the medical field; especially in his/her speciality of practice. This philosophy of continuous lifelong learning of doctors helps in improving effective healthcare delivery.

**Definition:** Lifelong learning initiative: "Lifelong learning is the progression and development of human potential by a continuously supportive process which empowers and provides impetus to a person in acquiring knowledge, values, skills, and understanding so as to successfully employ these with confidence and creativity in all arising circumstances and changing environments during course of his/her lifetime in the profession he/she practices".

## NEEDS AND SCOPE

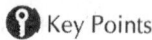 Key Points

1. **For self-assessment of their knowledge and skills:** In order to keep pace with recent advances in medical field, the doctors realize their strength and weaknesses in practice by difficulty and ease they face while diagnosis and management of clinical cases and thus they are able to recognize an objective self-assessment of their knowledge and skills and this gives them an impetus to continue learning and updating and upgrading their existing knowledge and skills and thus they acquire new skills.

2. **For employing gained knowledge in clinical practice:** An efficient physician employs his/her gained knowledge and skills in treatment and management of patients. Thus, it reflects their potential of introspection and utilization of experiences, in promoting and enhancement of their personal knowledge and thereby enhancing their professional growth and learning.

3. **For keeping update with recent advances:** The doctors employ various techniques in updating their knowledge and these include participation in continue medical education program, seminars and symposium on recent advances in their speciality, attending and presenting papers in conferences, use of digital media and Medlar Medline online libraries search engines by internet browsing, reading latest journals and books, and also by enrolling in short-term or long-term medical academic programs run by universities/health organizations.

4. **For choosing a career pathway:** A characteristic trait of lifelong learning of medical education eventually helps in to recognize and choose a suitable career pathway which shall be professionally rewarding and personally fulfilling his/her academic goals.

5. **For employing the changed dynamics of the patient healthcare:** The advancement in scientific technology and innovations (example: telemedicine and employing artificial intelligence) makes it essential for physicians (doctors) to upgrade to understand and imbibe the changed dynamics of the patient healthcare and its delivery.

6. **For matching local area healthcare needs:** The physicians also must match the local area healthcare needs depending on the disease prevalent in those areas, as well they should be aware of innovation in machinery-methodology of investigative protocols and modified treatment regime of diseases, and state and nation's legislative initiatives (applicable laws, consumer protection acts) and therefore arise the need and necessity of constant lifelong updating of knowledge for physician.

7. **For effective communication and discussion with fellow doctors:** Treatment in chain—the treatment protocol of a chain of doctors involved in management as seen in multispeciality hospitals (physician, neurologist, cardiologist, radiologist, pathologist, etc.) makes doctors self-conscious to keep update with knowledge of the day, as they are constantly

interacting with each other for effective healthcare delivery. Old days' single doctor–patient management care is gradually waning off.

8. **For employing standard of patients' heathcare treatment protocol:** The concept of health analytics in effective health practices has made need for healthcare benefit assessment more necessary as the increasing data sets available in open web domain which are becoming standard for patients' healthcare evaluation has thus warranted need by physicians to gain and update adequate knowledge of statistics and interpretation as a part of lifelong learning.

9. **For updating with changing medical laws and ethics:** The ethics guidelines in clinical practices are constantly upgraded and amended [examples: MTP (medical termination of pregnancy) Act, Organ Donation Act, etc.] hence it has become must for physicians to update their knowledge in this relevance.

## IMPORTANCE

1. **Lifelong learning reflects person's behaviour and personality:** An optimistic person always seeks for knowledge and being self-motivated enhances his/her knowledge and skills; as his/her personality traits are so.

2. **Self-learning or learning at workplace:** This is an important mode of active interactive learning by discussing with your senior professionals, peers and supervisors.

3. **It helps in personal career progression through performance appraisals by superiors and inputs from colleagues:** This stands as a very appropriate assessment for self-improvement unless some workplace biases exist in organization.

4. **Evidence-based practice and learning:** It helps in making sensible decisions by analysing the choicest patient-oriented evidence with patient-centred care available via research evidences and meta-analysis.

## CONCLUSION

Lifelong learning helps to gain confidence in practice, moreover the application of newly gained knowledge and skills is helpful in managing patient and moreover the updated knowledge is supportive of best evidence-based healthcare delivery outcomes which have been analysed and studied by the lifelong progressive learners. The physician's moral is higher if he/she is well versed with recent advances and can guide the work-force under him/her with confidence and commitment. He/she may also apply recent advancement and innovation in reference to machinery methodology and techniques in patient's management.

## ROLE OF A PHYSICIAN IN HEALTHCARE SYSTEM

### INTRODUCTION

The physician's primary role is to treat and manage diseases, health, educates his/her patients, relatives and the health staff, participates in implementing national health programs and contributes towards preventive and prophylaxis management especially in epidemics and prevention of spreading of communicable diseases.

**Key Points**

1. **Role as team leader:** The physician has multiple responsibilities as team leader and plays a diverse role in coordinating, directing, staffing, communicating, supervising, and imparting effective healthcare delivery.

2. **Treatment and management of disease:** The principal role of a physician is treating and managing the disease of his/her patients.

3. **Catering heath delivery:** His/her role is of primary importance in catering effective healthcare delivery in primary (primary health centres at village level), secondary (at district level hospitals) and tertiary healthcare (in municipality and city hospitals referral centres) settings.

4. **Role in health education:** The physician's role as health educator is of prime importance as he/she provides knowledge and helps in sharpening the skills of the work-force (paramedics, nurses, technicians, multipurpose workers, etc.) and other members of the medical healthcare team and this helps in maximizing the potential work output indirectly helping in providing best medical healthcare.

5. **Role as promoter of health economics and of social entrepreneur:** The physician while serving the society, utilizes the healthcare system and health delivery in an appropriate, cost-effective manner in concurrence with the national healthcare policies and thus ensures economically viable healthcare delivery preventing wastage of government expenditures.

6. **Role in generating healthcare data:** The physician's services are based on ability to collect, analyse and utilize health data and available statistics effectively. A physician may conduct survey and community-based statistical research to evaluate benefits of healthcare delivery, similarly these data may serve as information for planning future healthcare strategies.

7. **Role in prevention of diseases:** The physician employs preventive measure strategies to prevent spreading (communicating) of diseases in the community. He/she promotes and recommends lifestyle changes in management of diseases.

8. **Role in improving quality of life and lifespan:** The physician by providing therapeutic, curative, preventive and rehabilitative services reduces health burden in community, and thereby improves human quality of life and lifespan.

9. **Role in management of epidemics:** Epidemics of contagious diseases may be life-threatening and timely management and awareness (health education) by doctors can help in reducing risk of catastrophic situations as in epidemics.

10. **Role as a behavioural therapist in community:** The physician practicing with humanistic approach (treating with compassion and care) helps building-in trust in patients and this has found to be effective in developing confidence, solace and optimistic hope in patient, thus this behavioural approach hastens recovery. This doctor–patient trust in community members (as a medical practitioner is usually family doctor of many in the society) stands as behavioural therapy approach in community-based healthcare.

11. **Role in building professionalism and respect towards doctor community:** The professionalism in practices by doctors such as abiding by codes of ethics establishes high ethical standards and this helps in looking forwards towards doctors with respect, trust and confidence by community members thus establishing medical profession at high esteem in the community.

12. **Role as trainers of present and future generation of doctors for community:** The physicians provide on job training in teaching as well as service hospitals thus are developing manforce for future healthcare delivery. This also helps in improving the standard of patient care.

13. **Role as authoritative sources on clinical standards:** The physicians continue lifelong learning to update their medical knowledge thus they are looked forward as authoritative sources on clinical standards and practice for diagnosis and management by the community members for seeking consultation if required.

14. **Participation in national healthcare program:** The physician participates in implementing various national healthcare programs in community such as family welfare program, national tuberculosis management program, national program for prevention of malaria, leprosy, tuberculosis, etc.

15. **Participating as social workers:** The physician especially provides honorary services in shelter homes, home for the aged, slums, prison, or as a health provider NGO, etc. and thus provides social service to the community.

16. **Role in changing dynamics of the patient healthcare:** The advancement in scientific technology and innovations (e.g. telemedicine and employing artificial intelligence) makes it essential for physicians to upgrade to understand and imbibe the changed dynamics of the patient healthcare and its delivery.

17. **Provides services matching local area healthcare needs:** The physicians also must match the local area healthcare needs depending on the disease prevalent in those areas, innovation in machinery methodology of investigative protocols and modified treatment regime of diseases, and state and nations legislative initiatives (applicable laws, Consumer Protection Acts).

*Note: The students should note that the 'Role of physician in healthcare system' and 'Role of physician towards society and community' are synonymous, and in the next topic physician's role is completely discussed based on his/her role in society and towards community.*

## ROLE OF A PHYSICIAN TOWARDS SOCIETY AND COMMUNITY

🔑 Key Points

The principal role played by the physician towards society and community are as below:

1. **Medical expert:** The physician's primary role is diagnosing and treating the patients in the society. He/she identifies the speciality needed for the treatment and advices accordingly. He may advice the institutions, health bodies and state regarding required intervention in community health programs.

2. **Health communicator at community level:** Role in health education— the physician's role as educator is of prime importance as he provides knowledge and helps in sharpening the skills of the work-force (paramedics, nurses, technicians, multipurpose workers, etc.) and other members of the medical healthcare team and this helps.

3. **Role as collaborator at community level:** The physician should regularly attend CME, conferences and workshop and should exchange knowledge and skill gained with professional colleagues regionally and nationally.

4. **Role as community administrator and social entrepreneur:** The physician while serving the society, utilizes the healthcare system and health delivery in an appropriate, cost-effective manner in concurrence with the national healthcare policies and thus ensures economically viable healthcare delivery preventing wastage of government expenditures.

5. **Role as planner for future healthcare strategies in society:** The physician's health analytics are based on ability to collect, analyse and utilize health data and available statistics effectively. A physician may conduct survey and community-based statistical research to evaluate benefits of healthcare delivery, similarly these data may serve as information for planning future healthcare strategies in the society.

6. **Role as social and preventive medicine care provider:** The physician employs preventive measure strategies to prevent spreading (communicating) of diseases in the community. He/she promotes and recommends lifestyle changes in management of diseases.

7. **Role in improving quality of life and lifespan of community:** The physician employs preventive measure strategies to prevent spreading (communicating) of diseases in the community. He/she promotes and recommends lifestyle changes in management of diseases.

8. **Role as a behavioural therapist in community:** The physician practicing with humanistic approach (treating with compassion and care) helps

building-in trust in patients and this has found to be effective in developing confidence, solace and optimistic hope in patient, thus this behavioural approach hastens recovery. This doctor–patient trust in community members (as a medical practitioner is usually family doctor of many in the society) stands as behavioural therapy approach in community-based healthcare.

9. **Role in building professionalism and respect towards doctor community:** The professionalism in practices by doctors such as abiding by codes of ethics establishes high ethical standards and this helps in looking forwards towards doctors with respect, trust and confidence by community members thus establishing medical profession high esteem in the community.

10. **Role as trainers of present and future generation of doctors for community:** The physicians provide on job training in teaching as well as service hospitals thus are developing man-force for future healthcare delivery. This also helps in improving the standard of patient care.

11. **Role as scholar and health advocate:** The physicians continue lifelong learning to update their medical knowledge, thus they are looked forward as authoritative sources on clinical standards and practice for diagnosis and management by the community members for seeking consultation if required. The patient may approach a physician with local health issue and physician can work as health advocate to convey community request to local/state administration.

## Assignments for Evaluation

1. Discuss the professional qualities of physician.
2. Discuss the need, scope and importance of lifelong learning by physician.
3. Discuss the role of physician towards healthcare delivery.
4. Discuss the role of physician towards society and community.

## Short Answer Questions

1. What are the qualities of a good doctor?
2. Enlist qualities of a good physician.
3. Enlist importance for lifelong learning by the physician.
4. Discuss the lifelong learning methodologies for a doctor.
5. Discuss the role of a physician as a behavioural therapist.
6. Enlist few national health programs in which a physician is expected to participate.

7. How can a physician build professionalism and command respect towards doctor community?

8. How can a physician accommodate to changing dynamics of patient healthcare?

9. How is a physician involved in generating healthcare data?

10. Enlist the role of a physician towards society and community?

_____

_____

_____

_____

_____

_____

_____

_____

_____

_____

_____

_____

_____

_____

_____

_____

_____

_____

_____

_____

_____

_____

_____

_____

_____

## EXERCISE FOR STUDENTS

### SESSION I

### Exploratory Session (2 hours)

A lecture session addressing the competency can be followed by a small group discussion.

Arrange a small group discussion exploring the mindset of students regarding reasons for choosing medical profession, their perception regarding privileges and the responsibilities of the doctor and medical profession. What are their future goals and commitment for service towards the society?

**Reflections:** The students should note the key points of the lecture and summarise the knowledge gained by them.

_____

_____

_____

_____

_____

_____

_____

_____

_____

_____

_____

_____

_____

_____

_____

_____

_____

_____

## SESSION II

### Symposium Panel Discussion

A symposium cum panel discussion can be arranged for students where doctors of various specialities shall discuss regarding their experience in medical profession.

**Reflections:** The student should note the key points of various speakers on the occasion.

## SESSION III

### Self-directed Learning

The students should explore the text, notes of panel discussion, newspapers, books, research articles, inspirational movie for learning the topic.

**Reflections:** The students should note the activities conducted by them as summary.

**SESSION IV**

## Introductory Visit to the Hospital (2 Hours)

OPD, wards, labs, rehabilitation unit, medical record section, laundry, canteen, blood bank, etc.

**Reflections:** The student should comprehend the hospital visit as a report of about 250 words.

_____

_____

_____

_____

_____

_____

_____

_____

_____

_____

_____

_____

_____

_____

_____

_____

_____

_____

_____

_____

_____

_____

_____

_____

_____

**SESSION V**

## Comprehension and Conclusion

a. The student may be instructed to present the knowledge gained after completion of Module 1.1 in small groups.

b. A white coat ceremony may be arranged for students during the session.

**Reflections:** The students should take a brief note of the activities conducted during the session.

_____

_____

_____

_____

_____

_____

_____

_____

_____

_____

_____

_____

_____

_____

_____

_____

_____

_____

_____

_____

_____

_____

_____

_____

_____

# ENACT A ROLE-PLAY DEPICTING PARENTS' DREAM AND YOUR DREAM, EXPECTATION AND ACHIEVEMENT IN ENTERING INTO MEDICAL PROFESSION

## SAMPLE SCRIPT

### Parents' Dream

This is dream of millions of youngsters preparing for the premedical entrance test so was it for Abhishek and Annupriya.

Medical being a most respectable and noble profession, it is a dream of many parents to see their children become doctors not only for fame and money but for serving the community and humanity too.

It is one of the local trains in Mumbai and travellers from Navi Mumbai boarding the train at 8 am are busy chatting around .....

**Mr Deshpande:** Namaskar Chowdry Saheb: How is life?

**Mr Chowdry:** Nothing real friend, just busy with my son's coaching for medical entrance.

**Mr Deshpande:** Oh, it's same here, my daughter Annupriya is also trying her best for NEET and AIIMS entrance exams.

**Mr Chowdry:** That's good.

Next station arrives where Mr Banarjee and Mr Iyer both officers with State Bank of India join Mr Chowdry and Mr Deshpande who are the regular co-passengers from Suburb to Chhatrapati Shivaji Terminus (CST).

**Mr Chowdry:** Hi Mr Banerjee, have your son filled the PMT entrance exam form for AIIMS, New Delhi?

**Mr Banerjee:** Well yes and Shantanu is really engaged with medical entrance coaching for 8 hours/day.

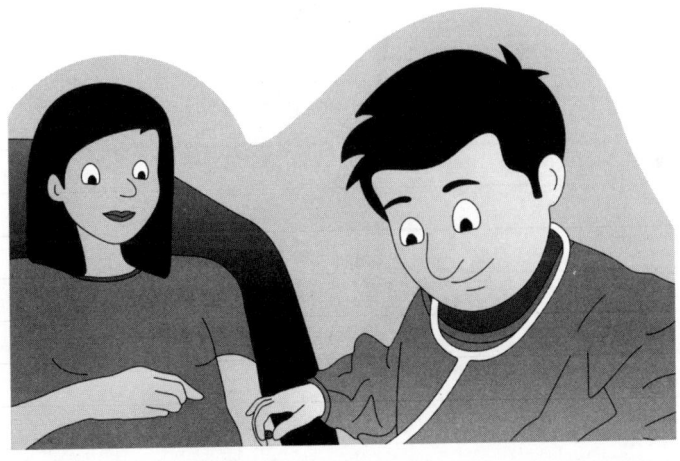

**Mr Iyer:** Friends, which is the best medical college to aim for?

**Mr Banerjee:** As per ranking made by some newspapers AIIMS New Delhi stands first, second is AFMC Pune, third is CMC Vellore and fourth is JIPMER Pondicherry, but this ranking changes every year but all said and done studying from government medical college is something good.

**Mr Iyer:** But my daughter Malini is a mediocre student and is planning to join any private medical college preferably under state or central university. Deemed university has its own pros and cons.

One fellow passenger introduces herself as Mrs Poonam Verma starts conversing...

**Mrs Poonam Verma:** I heard that fees in private medical colleges are very high approximately 1 crore for the 5 years of study. Is it really worth the expenditure?

**Mrs Jaspreet Arora:** A school principal in the next chair to Poonam exclaims: That's worth the bargain; my nephew who did MBBS MD from KEM is now settled in London and married a MRCOG gynaecologist from Ludhiana. They are minting money like anything.

**Another co-passenger:** Mrs Kulkarni, office clerk with PWD: My brother's son is a leading cardiologist practicing in Pune and his wife a radiologist. Both have made it great in career and are having many mansions.

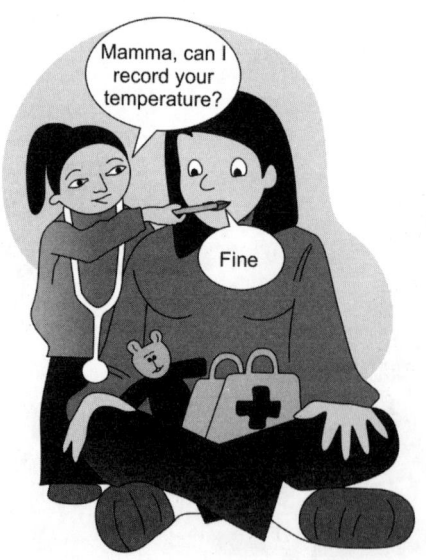

**Mrs Jaspreet Arora:** My daughter Tina has completed her MBBS from Lady Hardings, New Delhi and has cleared her USMLE part I and waiting for her Residency posting in US.

**Mr Iyer:** It is time to get down, all the best for the day friends. Whispers of bye... bye... as the group gets down at CST.

Whether it is Mumbai Chowpathy or Marina beach Chennai, or is busy bus travellers of Kolkata or Chat at teastalls of Banaras; the dream of Aaam Admi—can my child become a doctor?

## PREMEDICAL ENTRANCE EXAMINATION

The story behind the hardwork, dedication and devotion to clear medical entrance is not that easy. The dreams of parents start from toddlers where parents aspiring medical profession for the children purchase doctor's set a play toy when child is of 2 years.

The Grand Pa and Grand Ma reminds him/her at every play time—"Munna bada doctor bannega; Hamari Munni badi doctorni hogi".

HSSC board exams are over and students are rushing to NEET centres to have a last go through at one of the leading centres in New Delhi.

**Abhishek:** I have completed two revisions of test notes, revised over my CBSE textbooks for tenth time, since I started my preparation for PMT after passing my SSC exam.

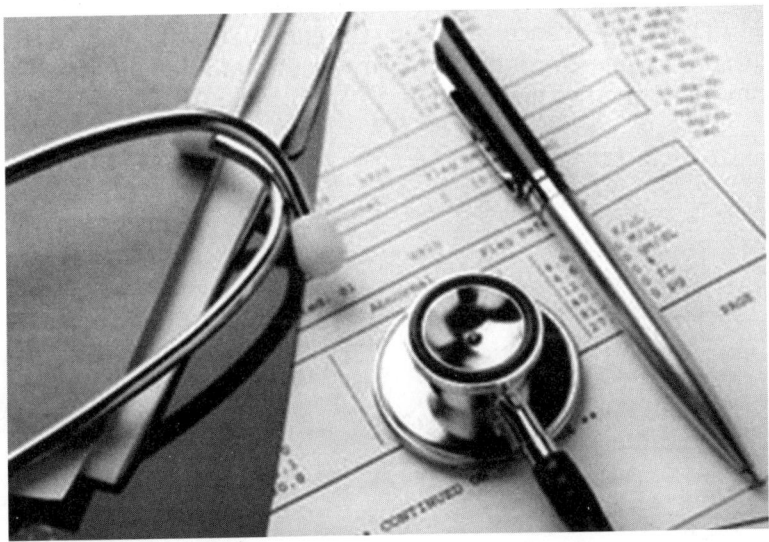

**Anurag:** I have completed reading and memorising the NCERT textbooks for XI and XII standards.

**Shanti:** I hope boys you have practiced solving the multiple choice questions in addition to that I have updated myself with general knowledge questions referring the latest books.

**Kokila:** Well Shanti you had been a cat throughout your career!

**Mousmi:** I wish, I will get through AIIMS entrance exams.

**Radhika:** Friends, I want to serve Indian Army and am mainly targeting for entering AFMC Pune.

**Ranjan:** Radhika—you have to clear the interview too for AFMC.

**Dinesh:** For me JIPMER will be the best since my maternal home town is Puducherry.

**Rajesh:** I will prefer any good medical college anywhere.

**Marina:** I will be in Kerala; many of my seniors have done well in PMT after being trained in Thrissur PMT study centre.

**Subramaniam:** Madras Medical College is my choice, well Stanley or Kilpauk Medical College will be fine too. I have to score centum in XII board exam and my dreams are through.

**Subhashish:** Any government medical college in Kolkata will be too good for me.

There are lakhs of students appearing for few thousand seats in medical colleges. Elite class parents prefer booking MBBS seats 2 to 3 years in advance; by paying the annual package about a crore or so. Dreams come true and joy in the families of successful candidates knows no bound.

# What does it Mean to be a Patient?

*Maria Pauline*

## Competencies Addressed

*The student should be able to:*

1. Enumerate and describe professional qualities and roles of a physician
2. Demonstrate empathy in patient encounters

## ▌Learning Experience

### An exploratory session (2 hours)

This session may be conducted as a continuous two hours session that may be split into two parts or as two one hour sessions, thereby giving time to the students to reflect on the discussion conducted in the first session and come up with their own specific examples of either personal ill health or that of a close family member or friend.

## SESSION 1

The instructor can start the session by introducing the concepts of empathy and equanimity in the context of the role of a doctor who helps patients, who are ill with associated suffering. Since these concepts are related to what we perceive as the role of a doctor, the instructor may need to explain the basic cardinal roles that a doctor needs to fulfill.[1] Following this, the instructor may ask students for their viewpoint on what their role may be when they become qualified as doctors.

Empathy is a key component of the patient-doctor encounter. Coming from the doctor, it helps the patient to lower his/her defensiveness enough to let the doctor know about his/her needs. This enables the doctor to be able to gauge the environment of the patient that might help or hinder with the treatment modalities;

this leads to better accuracy of diagnosis and higher chances of the effectiveness of treatment.[2]

On the other end of the spectrum, equanimity or stoicism is another quality that the doctor needs to develop and use appropriately to enhance the effectiveness of patient-doctor encounters. Such equanimity becomes an essential tool for the doctor to be able to take clinical decisions without getting bogged down by difficult emotions, either on the part of the doctor, the patient or their caregivers.[3]

After introducing these core concepts of empathy, equanimity and detached concern, the instructor can then move onto real-life, blended or imaginary case studies to discuss these concepts with the students.

*A few such cases are described below.*

1. Three resident doctors of Mumbai hospital attacked by dead patient's kin.

   Press Trust of India, Mumbai. July 15, 2019 UPDATED: July 15, 2019 00:01 IST

   Three resident doctors of the civic-run Nair Hospital in central Mumbai were attacked on Sunday evening by kin of a patient, who died during treatment.

   Weblink: https://www.indiatoday.in/india/story/3-resident-doctors-mumbai-hospital-attacked-dead-patient-kin1569018-2019-07-15 2.

2. Patient's kin attack doctor at Hyderabad hospital IANS, Hyderabad. Last Updated at May 20, 2019 15:26 IST

   Relatives of a patient attacked a doctor at Nizam's Institute of Medical Sciences (NIMS) here in the early hours of Monday over his alleged negligence. Weblink: https://www.business-standard.com/article/ news-ians/patient-s-kin-attack-doctor-at-hyderabad-hospital119052000746_1.html

3. Kin of a patient who attacked junior resident doctor at Kolkata hospital to be charged with attempt to murder.

   Updated Jul 11, 2019 | 01:28 IST | Mirror Now Digital Close to a month after Dr Paribaha Mukherjee, a junior resident doctor at Kolkata's Nil Ratan Sircar (NRS) Medical College and Hospital, was attacked by relatives of a 75-year-old patient, a court in Sealdah city of West Bengal has now given police officials the permission to include Section 307 of the IPC which prescribes the punishment for attempt to murder.

Weblink: https://www.timesnownews.com/mirror-now/ crime/article/kin-of-patient-who-attacked-junior-resident- 56 Aetcom doctor-at-kolkata-hospital-to-be-charged-with-attempt-tomurder/451912 4.

4. A woman of Mumbai gets Rs 15 lakh payout 9 years after husband's death in 'medical negligence' case.

   Press Trust of India, Mumbai. Published: 02nd August 2019 12:21 PM | Last Updated: 02nd August 2019 12:21 PM.

   The state consumer commission in Maharashtra has directed a civic-run hospital in Navi Mumbai and a Chemburbased hospital to pay over Rs 15 lakh compensation to a woman whose husband died 9 years ago due to "medical negligence". In a recent order, the Maharashtra State Consumer Disputes Redressal Commission said while one hospital could not recognise the illness of her husband, the other did not provide proper medical treatment to him. Weblink:http://www. newindianexpress.com/cities/ kolkata/2019/aug/02/ mumbai-woman-gets-rs-15-lakhpayout-nine-years-after-husbands-death-in-medicalnegligence-case-2013051.html

5. A senior doctor of Bihar suspended for negligence as encephalitis death toll rises to 109 at Muzaffarpur hospital.

   India Today Web Desk, New Delhi. June 23, 2019 UPDATED: June 23, 2019 11:23 IST.

   A senior doctor from Sri Krishna Medical College and Hospital (SKMCH) in Muzaffarpur in Bihar has been suspended for negligence after 109 children admitted with acute encephalitis syndrome (AES) or Japanese encephalitis died due to lack of treatment.

   Weblink: https://www.indiatoday.in/india/story/biharsenior-doctor-suspended-for-negligence-as-encephalitisdeath-toll-rises-to-109-in-muzaffarpur-hospital-1554429-2019-06-23 6.

6. Too few doctors, too many patients in Calcutta hospitals.

   By Kinsuk Basu in Calcutta. Published 29.06.19, 4:37 AM. Updated 29.06.19, 4:37 AM.

   The NRS Medical College and Hospital, where two interns were attacked on the night of June 10 2019 after the death of a 75-year-old patient there, has only 1,886 beds. On Friday, more than 3,500 patients were in the inpatient wards. The head injury unit at NRS has 27 beds. On Friday, the last patient admitted was on trolley and had the serial number 111.

   Weblink: https://www.telegraphindia.com/states/westbengal/too-few-doctors-too-many-patients-in-calcuttahospitals/cid/1693422

## EXERCISE FOR STUDENTS

The students should record the lecture notes and cases discussed by them in exploratory session.

_____

_____

_____

_____

_____

_____

_____

_____

_____

_____

_____

_____

_____

_____

_____

_____

_____

_____

_____

_____

_____

_____

_____

_____

_____

## SESSION 2

For this session, the instructor could divide the students into groups, if dealing with a large class. Each group could be asked to present to the rest of the class one-two cases where either a student or their close family or friends were a patient. After each presentation, the instructor could initiate a discussion where the rest of the class pitches in with ideas of what they would have done different as (a) patients to have better coped with their ill health through improved interaction with their doctor and (b) doctor to have helped their patient cope better with the illness or its outcome. This session could be concluded with the instructor asking the student groups to write up the cases they presented and the ideas for alternative coping skills and strategies on patients' and doctors' part suggested by the rest of the class in the form of a report.

### EXERCISE FOR STUDENTS

The students should record the topics and cases discussed by them in small group discussion session.

_____

_____

_____

_____

_____

_____

_____

_____

_____

_____

_____

_____

_____

_____

_____

_____

_____

_____

_____

_____

_____

_____

_____

_____

_____

_____

_____

_____

_____

_____

_____

_____

_____

_____

_____

_____

_____

_____

_____

_____

_____

_____

_____

## REFERENCES

1. Godlee F. The role of the doctor. *BMJ: British Medical Journal* 2007; 335 (7628), 0.
2. Mercer SW, Reynolds WJ, Empathy and quality of care. *Br J Gen Pract* 2002; 52 (Suppl), S9–12.
3. Halpern J. What is clinical empathy? *Journal of General Internal Medicine* 2003; 18(8), 670–674.

## Short Answer Questions

1. What is the role of a doctor?
2. What is clinical empathy?
3. As a doctor, if you had to choose between empathy and equanimity toward your patients, which one would you choose and why?
4. Will your choice, as a doctor, between empathy and equanimity toward a patient depend on (a) the patient's socioeconomic status and (b) cause of the illness: Patient action driven (smoking for example) versus circumstantial (heavy metal exposure during mining)? Explain your position.
5. How will you interact with a patient or their caregiver to inform them about a clinical complication that has arisen due to negligence or mistake on your part or of the hospital?
6. What suggestion(s) would you come up with for a hospital to empathetically and consciously manage interaction with patients and their caregivers in cases where clinical complications have arisen due to negligence or mistake on part of the attending doctors or nurses or other hospital staff?
7. Would you be comfortable treating your close friends or family members? Should there be guidance or training in medical colleges for such interactions?
8. Should hospitals institute recording of patient feedback on doctors' quality of interacting with the patients, especially in specializations such as psychiatry, paediatrics and HIV clinics? Explain your stand.
9. Assuming a high patient load per doctor in low socioeconomic areas, which of the following should be prioritized—number of patients treated or the time spent per patient treated to maximize health outcomes?

SESSION II

Symposium: Panel Discussion

A symposium cum panel discussion can be arranged for students where doctors of various specialities share their experiences during their

to discuss their opinions, views, etc. on the topic as moderated by the medium of the discussion.

## EMPATHY IN PATIENT ENCOUNTERS

Throughout the world, the impact of advances in medicine has brought in significant implications in the management of patients by the healthcare givers. Gradually, as members of diverse specialties recognize the clinical, ethical and societal attitudes, the relevance to diagnosis and treatment, takes a different perspective in their routine clinical practice.

In our healthcare system that rewards procedures more than talking with our patients, the communication skills and time required for effective counselling, providing information and an 'empathetic' attitude towards achieving the patients goal is forgotten.

A rational framework is required from student days to incorporate these attitudes among medical professional to bring about a connectedness between the patient and doctor. Several reports have now proved that competency is not only proved by their qualifications but by their 'warmth' which is displayed to their patients.

An integral part of this training for medical students would involve teaching and training them the essentials of good communication skills, rapport building and exercises which allow them to reflect on the changing scenario of patient-doctor interaction.

Empathy is often defined as an individual capacity, as his/her capacity to place oneself in another's position, which entails a social-emotional ability to be more affective, i.e. the ability to share the emotions of others, and cognitive, i.e. the ability to understand the emotions of others.

As per our Graduate Medical Education Regulations, 2017— Global Attitude, Ethics and Communication Competencies are addressed in the roles of an Indian Medical Graduate and physician's empathy is essential to patient centered care. Overall the physician based emphatic approach to the patient's situation is often linked to increased patient satisfaction, adherence, patient comprehension, patient perception of a good interpersonal relationship and thereby improving the health status of the patient.

Although more often in medical education verbal communication is emphasized more than non-verbal communication, empathy forms an important component of non-verbal communication. A holistic and humane concern for patient well-being thus drives home the standard for care forward and incentives for quality healthcare.

Finally we need to bring about a balance, between our knowledge (professionalism) and communication (ethics). Our words can either facilitate or complicate our communication. By reinforcing our integrity and consistency in counselling the patients, we need to consider all the consequences and repercussions such information may have on the patient. Further research on the psychosocial and ethical implications of medical information are needed to formulate policies to meet the patient's need as individuals, members of families, communities and the society.

## STUDENT'S ROLE

Clinical empathy, often described as the physicians' emotional attunement to serve the cognitive goal of understanding patients' emotions are difficult to convey and envisage in the initial years of medical training, as it overrides the vast and increasing medical knowledge. Ideally during a conversation between the patient and doctor both professionalism and empathy need to be maintained to make the counselling session effective.

While training our students in the art of medicine, we need to build a foundation based on knowledge and experience when they relate to the patients. There are several ways in which a student can imbibe this skill of communication. Clinical orientation programs can be conducted soon after their first year to offer an early clinical exposure to their clinical postings.

These programs are meant to give them a first-hand exposure to the practices of clinical medicine by observing the senior doctors in the management and counselling/interaction with the patients.

For example, when parents whose child has a mental and physical disability come for counselling, in an attempt to explore the possibility of having a normal child in the future pregnancy: Several factors are to be taken into consideration in identifying the cause of the first child's condition. Once the proper diagnosis and investigations are done and ascertained, the counselling process is done over periodic sessions. During these sessions several factors are revealed and non-verbal behaviour implicated by the doctor's empathy is a tremendous task. The empathetic and professional attitudes need to be maintained throughout all sessions. It is very important to be sensitive to the problems being faced by parents of a disabled child. Often parents can break down in front of the doctor and express their problems and fears.

Awareness into the medical, social, cultural, economic and personal aspects of interaction with the patient allows an insight to the scenario in a clinic. Discussions and role playing, is another aspect which students can relate to and helps them to understand empathic responses which result from the interaction between behavioural and emotional factors.

Another important attribute is being a 'good listener'. Every patient wants to be treated as person and not as an illness, which increases the responsibility of the doctor to respond empathically.

The actual emotional process of empathy may also be aided by exercises such as self-reflective writing, which helps an observer become more aware of his/her own emotions and subsequently improve his/her ability to be empathetic towards another.

These training sessions as well as bed side teaching should inculcate the values of personalized care and help the students to learn and become effective communicators and skilled physicians. It is imperative that we incorporate empathic non-verbal training into medical education. A recent meta-analysis shows that empathy trainings can be successful, by emphasizing non-verbal behaviour which shows a significant increase to patient ratings of clinician empathy. Striving toward professionalism may threaten healthcare quality unless self-assessment methods are encouraged to alter the empathy decline among trainees.

Empathy is an emotional identification of both heart and mind. Doctors who display empathic non-verbal behaviour—such as posture, eye contact, facial expression (smiling), touch and uncrossed arms—are perceived as both warmer and more competent.

"Our findings might reflect a changing concept of the role of doctors in our society. No longer are they judged solely on their technical competence—that is, their ability to perform medical procedures. Rather they may increasingly be judged on their interpersonal competence—that is, their ability to navigate the difficult social interactions inherent in managing patients' illness and wellness," wrote study author Gordon T. Kraft-Todd in a Scientific American blog.

Twenty years ago, no one was talking about the role of empathy and emotions in healthcare, and detachment was still part of the traditional formula for a good doctor. But now we know that the physician's empathy is known to be associated with positive health outcomes, increased diagnostic accuracy, more patient adherence to treatment and increased patient satisfaction. The literature suggests there are specific physician behaviours, both verbal and non-verbal, that increase the probability that a patient will perceive the physician as caring.

Very often we need to employ and preserve cognitive empathy, even when affective empathy (sympathy) may decline, so that you can actually learn the things that are going to help your patients. Even gender of the doctor plays a role for a satisfactory doctor–patient relationship. Studies have proved that female doctors show more empathy towards their patients compared to the male doctors.

In pursuit of this physician–patient interaction, the physician must project a genuinely caring attitude toward the patient, by being reflective in response to an observed feeling or emotion, being non-judgmental about their experiences and validate or legitimize their reflection by willing to understand these emotional reaction of their patients.

For example, in the case of a child recently diagnosed with juvenile diabetes mellitus type 1. The clinical skills in interviewing the parents, examination and building a rapport with the patient and his/her parents to understand the situation, provides a 'connection' to the relationship between the doctor and patient. Management and follow up becomes more satisfying, reflecting a genuine care for the welfare of the patient.

In response to this attribute, the doctors who are more aware of their patients' emotional needs and respond appropriately to their concerns feel satisfied with their jobs, experience less stress, cynicism, and burnout than those with less empathy.

According to the Empathic Communication Coding System (ECCS) explicit recognition of the patient's perspective is central to the communication of empathy. In conclusion, it is imperative that human interaction is characterized by mutuality of linguistic alignment, reciprocal adjustments, synchrony of movements, and psychophysiological processes. Thus, empathic communication is essential to progress in the interrelated realms of medical education, practical research, and patient care.

## Short Answer Questions

1. What is clinical empathy? Is it essential in present doctor–patient relationship?
2. To what extent should physician respond to empathic opportunities?
3. In your opinion what are the factors involved in the level of empathy to the patient–doctor relationship?
4. Do medical students benefit from an early clinical exposure before starting their clinical postings and how far are empathetic responses important in their training?

# Doctor–Patient Relationship

*K Rajgopal Shenoy*

### Competencies Addressed
*The student should be able to:*
1. Enumerate and describe professional qualities and roles of a physician
2. Demonstrate empathy in patient encounters

### ▌ Learning Objective Background

The students after learning this module, should be able to describe and discuss the
1. Professional qualities of doctors and their duties.
2. Empathy experienced while treating patient.
3. Fundamentals of doctor–patient relationship and issues associated with ethics in relevance to duties and responsibility of a doctor.

Referring to the work of physicians, Dr Elmer Hess, a former President of the American Medical Association, once wrote: "There is no greater reward in our profession than the knowledge that God has entrusted us with the physical care of His people. The Almighty has reserved for Himself the power to create life, but He has **assigned to a few of us the responsibility of keeping in good repair the bodies in which this life is sustained."** Accordingly, reverence for human life and individual dignity is both the hallmark of a good physician and the key to truly beneficial advances in medicine.

### INTRODUCTION

What is the need to write this chapter—doctor–patient relationship? The answer lies in the observation that litigations against doctors are becoming common. Doctors are being targeted often not only because of complications that happened during their treatment of patients but also because they do not have unity. Expectations of the patients are high and the reasons for litigations are many. Patients expect that doctors provide a complete and even miraculous cure. Patients and their relatives feel that the hospital and doctors have charged exorbitant fees but they did not get cured, developed complications or the patient has died. Patients are aware of consumer courts. Many lawyers are ready to support their clients and get them compensation. All these are facts. Complications are known to occur in spite of the best treatment. The main factor often missing in this entire scenario is the vital doctor–patient relationship. This article highlights the importance of a good rapport between the doctor and the patient. The following points are important not only to maintain doctor–patient relationship but also to decrease friction between the patient and the doctor.

**Attitude:** Attitude of a doctor towards the patient is the first step which builds a rapport between the two. When the patient is in pain and is suffering, identify the condition properly, treat it and console him/her. Rather than treat him/her like customer at a hotel or a shop, a humanitarian approach to make him/her comfortable would be much more appropriate and help build a good relationship.

**Benevolent:** A doctor should be gentle while receiving the patient and then examining the patient. He should have sympathy and understanding towards the patient. That does not mean that he should shed tears. The doctor should be kind-hearted, gracious, considerate and compassionate.

**Communication, competency and continued learning:** The doctor–patient relationship starts from the first visit of the patient to the doctor. The first impression is the best impression. Good communication skills impress. If we look back to 20–30 years ago, our family physicians did not even have MBBS degree, leave alone specialization and superspecialization. They were ready to listen to the patient, do home visits, attend midnight calls and accept whatever money that was given to them. Doctors were looked upon as Gods and patients accepted both success and failure. Their success was largely because of good communication skills. The world is changing at a great speed and moving ahead. Communication alone does not heal but good medical care is needed. Medicine is changing. We cannot sit idle without updating our knowledge. With continuous medical education, theoretical knowledge can be updated. One can improve skills by attending conferences and watching surgeries in workshops and thus attain competency. Patients also feel happy that the doctor has attended many conferences all over the world and has improved his knowledge.

**Dignity and diversity:** India is a country of multiple languages and many cultures. Diversity is our strength. The doctor should be sensitive to these cultural differences while treating the patients. Give respect to their culture and appreciate rather than discourage or argue. Our deeds should not have any deleterious effect on the body or mind.

**Evidence-based practice and ethics:** Every doctor should appreciate the need for update and be familiar with different therapeutic modalities, administration of 'essential drugs' and their common side-effects. The latest possible information should be passed on to the patient with scientific data so that he is aware of what is the best solution for the present problem. Knowledge is strength and that gives us confidence while talking to the patient or while attending the courts. While making the patient comfortable, it is not just enough to tell him what disease he has and what can be done. Convey the various options available and the cost of the treatment. Most often, problem arises because of inadequate information and options. Often the patient says, "Doctor, you do it". I still do open hernia repair but I tell my patients about laparoscopic hernia repair. Vast majority of patients agree to what you say. When you cannot do it or do not have facilities, it is better to refer to higher centres rather than provide substandard initial treatment.

**Family physician:** In the present times, a surgeon or physician cannot truly become a family physician because of specialization. However, we can have all the characteristics of a family physician. To name a few, patience to listen, smile on the face till late night clinic, enquiring about his professional life and family life. They really used to satisfy some important mission of doing MBBS, i.e. being competent to practice preventive, promotive, curative and rehabilitative medicine with respect to the commonly encountered health problems in a patient and in community.

**Help:** Call for help is the most important step in today's practice, especially when a surgical procedure is planned. It is vital to obtain a proper informed consent after explaining all possible complications to the patient.

**Conclusion:** Just look back at the Hippocratic Oath we took when we joined medical school (for me, 1977). How many of us remember the oath? We have worked hard to get the basic MBBS degree and then postgraduation. We acquired the basic knowledge to diagnose and manage common health problems of the individual and the community appropriate to his/her position as a member of the health team at primary, secondary and tertiary levels. We need to introspect about keeping our house neat. These are my final thoughts which are simple and common:

1. We must know and accept our limitations.
2. Refer patients on time, not late.
3. Communicate with patients and their families effectively.
4. Do what is required for the patient at the moment without commenting on the past or commenting on others' treatment.
5. Do not negate patient's views even after you convince effectively.
6. Don't react impulsively and adversely.
7. Be patient with your patients.
8. Do your job to satisfy your conscience.
9. Be united in critical times.
10. Keep yourself updated about your subject.

## Mutual Understanding and Trust between Patient and the Physician

A physician provides medical care to his/her patient and at times also provides moral solace and advises in case of emotionally disturbed patient. The patient and his/her relatives acknowledge the act of the doctor's good-will and his/her professional skills in attaining recovery in patient's health. Thus, whenever a patient comes to his/her physician, an unwritten contract binds the doctor towards his/her duty and patients towards expressing their gratitude and trust towards the doctor.

But question arises in case of litigation involving medical negligence even false complaints against doctors. Therefore, physician should abide by the ethical principles in clinical practice, obtain a written consent for any investigation and therapeutic procedures. He/she must maintain confidentiality to discuss and explain the treatments to be employed with patient or his/her relatives, seek second opinion if the condition warrants and ensures following the medical ethics meticulously to the core.

Thus to conclude, the physician should safeguard patient's confidence within the spheres of the laws of ethics. The physician under ethics should disclose the necessary information regarding patient's condition. The disclosure must be relevant to the situation and the physician must maintain privacy of the patient judiciously and in the interest of his/her welfare.

The physician should duly respect the law and also be willing to accept changes in the treatment modality in best interest of patient's health, if the condition warrants.

Thus a mutual trust and understanding under spheres of medical ethics between doctor and patient is helpful in providing effective healthcare.

**Note:** The students should note that the professional quality and role of physician have also been discussed in Module 1.2. The defined competency for Module 1.2 and Module 1.3 are same.

## ASSIGNMENT FOR STUDENTS

### Short Answer Questions

1. Discuss how attitude helps to build rapport with the patient?
2. How does a doctor exhibit benevolence while treating his/her patients?
3. How are communication, competency and continued learning helpful in building doctor–patient relationship?
4. Discuss the importance of dignity and diversity in management of patients?
5. What do you understand by evidence-based practice and ethics?
6. Discuss the role and importance of family physician.
7. What do you understand by concept of health for all?
8. Enlist the key elements necessary for a doctor to be a role model in society.

## EXERCISE FOR STUDENTS

### SESSION I

Exploratory session can be arranged for students in the form of interactive lecture (1 hour).

**Reflections:** The students should note the key points of lecture and discussion.

_____

_____

_____

_____

_____

_____

_____

_____

_____

_____

_____

_____

_____

_____

_____

_____

_____

_____

_____

_____

_____

_____

_____

## SESSION II

### Self-learning by Students (2 hours)

a. The students can be divided in groups. They can be provided with books/CD/DVD/newspapers on the topic for exploration and self-learning.

b. The students may be asked to present their learning achievement in small groups.

**Reflections:** The student should note the protocol of activities carried by them.

## SESSION III

A small group discussion (2 hours) can be coupled with debate, elocution, oral presentation, role play, etc.

**Reflections:** The students may record the key points of discussions and activities conducted by them.

_____

_____

_____

_____

_____

_____

_____

_____

_____

_____

_____

_____

_____

_____

_____

_____

_____

_____

_____

_____

_____

_____

_____

_____

_____

_____

_____

_____

## SESSION IV

Concluding session can be coupled with seminar presentation by students and case discussion. Four example case discussions are given below.

### Case Discussion 1

A 28-year-old male underwent appendicectomy following which his symptoms of abdominal pain subsided. After a week's time, the patient complained of intermittent intense pain and constipation. On examination, the abdomen was slightly tender and a mobile, rubbery mass of 18–20 cm was observed in the periumbilical area. The doctor suggested laparotomy procedure as line of management to the patient but the patient refused. The doctor got furious and asked the patient never to return for any consultation.

*Points for discussion:*

1. Harmony in doctor–patient relationship and trust factor.
2. The role and responsibility of the doctor and the patient's rights.
3. Is patient's request for second opinion, incorrect for termination of doctor–patient relationship?

### Case Discussion 2

A 50-year-old female patient was diagnosed to have uterine cancer stage III B (cancer had spread to vagina or the uterus).

The busy gynecologist planned for hysterectomy. The patient's relative wished to discuss the details and wanted to know the treatment modalities.

The gynecologist unwilling to spend time towards further counselling asked them to take the patient wherever they want and she would not treat her then.

*Discuss*

1. Was the doctor correct in her role of carrying out her duties?
2. Was it appropriate for the relatives to ask questions?
3. What should be the ideal doctor–patient communication in this case?

### Case Discussion 3

A patient reported to the doctor with a request to reissue his discharge card which he lost accidentally. The patient was very much concerned as the hospital discharge card mentioned his medical history, clinical profile, medication and follow-up treatment. The doctor refused to entertain his request due to his extremely busy schedule and instructed him to search for it at his residence. The patient got wild and argued with the doctor. The doctor furiously shoved the patient away and warned him not to come up with such request again.

1. Is doctor's conduct appropriate for the situation?
2. What should have been the doctor's attitude and response in the case?
3. Was patient's response appropriate or should he have waited for the doctor to be free from his primary duty of patient management?

### Case Discussion 4

A person injured in a scooter accident was brought to a private hospital in a critical condition. The consultant on duty had some urgent assignment outside. He instructed the patient's relative to take the patient to nearby government hospital and instructing the same to the nursing staff, he left the hospital.

1. What should have been the doctor's response in such situation?
2. What should be the standard protocol in management of critical cases in a hospital?

# The Foundations of Communication 1

*Sanjay Andrew Rajaratnam*

## Competencies Addressed

*The student should be able to:*

1. Demonstrate ability to communicate to patients in a patient, respectful, non-threatening, non-judgmental and empathetic manner.

## ■ Learning Objective Background

- Essential principles of communication for the health professional—an overview.
- Communicating with patients—the 5 A's behaviour change model.
- Communicating with patient—the Kalamazoo Consensus Statement.
- Communicating with patients—a case-based study on how doctors *must not* communicate.
- The doctor–patient communication—the way it must be.

## RECOMMENDED TEACHING-LEARNING METHODOLOGY

| Topic | Recommended teaching-learning method | Number of hours |
|-------|--------------------------------------|-----------------|
| Essential principles of communication for the health professional—an overview | Large group discussion | –Two– |
| Communicating with patients—the 5 A's behaviour change model | Small group discussion | –One– |

| | | |
|---|---|---|
| Communicating with patient—the Kalamazoo Consensus Statement | Small group discussion | –One– |
| Communicating with patients—a case-based study on how doctors *must not* communicate | Self-directed learning | –One and a half– |
| The doctor–patient communication—the way it must be | Student role play—supervised and corrected by a facilitator | –One and a half– |

## ESSENTIAL PRINCIPLES OF COMMUNICATION FOR THE HEALTH PROFESSIONAL—AN OVERVIEW

### ▮ Learning Objective Background

- Understand and define the word 'Communication' in the context of healthcare.
- Outline the landmarks of the communication process.
- Mention and summarize the types of communication in a healthcare set-up.
- Outline the barriers of communication in a healthcare set-up.
- Outline the facilitators of communication in a healthcare set-up.

**Communication—its implication to a health professional:** The word 'communication' refers to a meaningful exchange of thoughts, opinions or information between individuals belonging to any of the sectors of healthcare, e.g. doctors, patients, patient's families, nursing professionals or the administrators of healthcare.

Effective communication within the healthcare set-up fulfills the primary goal of healthcare, i.e. patient well-being and also prevents conflict between individuals that is often encountered in recent times.

**Landmarks of the communication process:** This can be understood as follows:

Communication begins from the **SENDER**, i.e. the primary source of information.

↓

**ENCODING** and **CHANNELING** of the information to be communicated refers to deciding and executing the mode by which the information is conveyed, i.e. through spoken words, written words or bodily gestures.

↓

**DECODING** and **RECEPTION** of the communicated information is the interpretation of the information communicated by the sender.

↓

**FEEDBACK** is a process of communication that points to the outcome of communication. Feedback may be formal, e.g. a questionnaire-based feedback or informal, e.g. a verbal feedback. Feedback of communication must be essentially obtained to strengthen the communication process in an environment.

## Types of Communication Encountered in a Healthcare Set-up:

Communication within a healthcare environment is depicted in the following Table.

| Communication based on the number of people involved in the process | Communication based on the medium used for the process | Communication based on the feedback obtained during the process | Communication directed by the authorities of an institute |
|---|---|---|---|
| 1. Intrapersonal communication | 1. Verbal communication | 1. Two-way communication | 1. Formal communication |
| 2. Interpersonal communication | 2. Non-verbal communication | 2. One-way communication | 2. Informal communication |
| 3. Group communication | | | |
| 4. Mass communication | | | |

*Intrapersonal communication* refers to the introspection or the self-reflection by the sender before he or she begins to communicate about a particular topic. This precedes *interpersonal communication* in which the communicator shares his or her opinion, drawn from intrapersonal communication, to one or more persons.

*Group communication* can be categorized as *large group communication*, e.g. a didactic lecture for 100 learners or *small group communication*, e.g. a small group discussion for 10 learners.

*Mass communication* is the communication directed to the society in general, e.g. through newspapers, television channels or electronic media.

*Verbal communication* specifically refers to spoken communication. On the other hand, *non-verbal communication* is a form of communication mediated by gestures, facial expressions or eye contact, to mention a few, in which the person who communicates gets his or her message across without using spoken words.

*Two-way communication* is a type of communication during which the message shared by the sender and the receiver is shared with the degree of understanding to be conveyed being achieved. This is the best form of communication in a healthcare set-up that overcomes misunderstanding and conflict. However, this form of communication may not be feasible in every circumstance.

*One-way communication* is a form of communication in which the message is passed on between the sender and receiver with the receiver being expected to execute the desired outcome of communication. In other words, this form of communication lacks feedback with the receiver being expected to mandatorily execute the communicated task. Only authoritative faculties of a working environment must carry out one-way communication after discussing the concerned matter adequately. If misused, this type of communication can lead to conflict and incompetence of the work executed.

*Formal communication* or vertical communication is an official communication within the institute that passes down from the highest level in the hierarchy of administration, e.g. institutional policies, notices or circulars relating to change. Grievances following this type of communication are usually communicated in an ascending order in the hierarchy of administration.

*Informal communication* is also known as horizontal communication. This type of communication refers to peer groups within an institute discussing their opinions on an event or task amongst themselves. This form of communication can lead to uncalled-for conflict and retardation of the working goal. However, at times, informal communication can refine a particular action taken by the hierarchy of administration towards better accomplishment of the working goal.

**Barriers to communication in the working environment:** This can be listed as follows.

1. Language barriers.
2. Cultural barriers.

3. Interpersonal barriers.
4. Erratic channeling of information.
5. Stereotyping.
6. Barriers due to perception of communicated information.
7. Physical barriers.
8. Emotional barriers.

*Language barriers* to communication in a healthcare set-up are quite often encountered in the working environment. To minimize this, the sender of information must be trained to memorize the commonly used phrases of the profession in the different languages spoken or encountered in the environment of work. If need be, a translator can be used to minimize this barrier to communication.

*Cultural barriers* to communication are commonly encountered in a healthcare set-up. This is addressed by the facilitators of healthcare being made to be aware of the different cultural attributes and using such knowledge to overcome them.

*Interpersonal barriers* that hinder communication are also commonly encountered in a healthcare set-up. This is overcome if the sender and receiver of information are focused on the primary goal of their duties while communicating.

*Erratic channeling of information* during communication can lead to misinterpretation with the desired outcome of the communication not being achieved. To prevent this barrier every employee of the institute must be aware of the corporate culture of the working environment.

*Stereotyping* of information during communication can result in a misperception of communication that a biased opinion is sent or received. Altering phrases while communicating a particular task minimizes this.

*Barriers due to perception of communicated information* are most often due to the sender and receiver of information being of different cultural backgrounds. It leads to misinterpretation of the communicated message. It can be minimized if the sender of information takes time to understand the person to whom the message is being delivered and clarifies issues that may lead to the message being misunderstood.

*Physical barriers* to communication in a working environment are space and noise. This is managed by the infrastructure of the working environment being adequately designed with appropriate management of overcrowding by the deputed personnel.

*Emotional barriers* during communication refer to either the sender or receiver of information being emotionally unstable due to being overworked. This is addressed by the time management of the working period of employees. Fear or worry during communication is another emotional barrier of communicating adequately. This is minimized by allowing time for the communicated message to be perceived correctly and not resorting to haste in this process.

**Facilitators of effective communication:** The desired outcome of communication can be facilitated by certain factors that a sender and receiver of information in a healthcare set-up must be aware of. These include:

1. Resorting to a positive attitude while communicating.
2. Timely updating of communication skills.
3. Acceptance and correction of miscommunication.
4. Keen listening of a communicated message.
5. Stating of defined objectives during communication.
6. Using the appropriate language while communicating.

*A positive approach* of the communication and/or sender of a message plays an important role in the communicated message being interpreted, as it must be. This in turn is mediated by factors mediating the communication process such as sincerity, trustworthiness, empathy, assertiveness, courtesy, warmth and self-confidence.

*Timely updating of communication skills* by healthcare personnel must be done. In current times, this can be done over the internet by updating the nuances of communication in a healthcare set-up in different healthcare centres around the world and implementing them if necessary in one's working environment. This, of course, must be done following a discussion with the administrators of the institute in concern.

*Acceptance and correction of miscommunication* can at times lead to conflict and this can be minimized if the sender and receiver of a message remember that no two individuals will perceive a communicated message exactly the way it should be with minimal differences in perception being bound to occur. This must be assessed and time must be allowed to correct the misperception of a communicated message.

*Keen listening of a communicated message* refers to the time taken to hear, interpret and understand communicated information. Time must be allowed for these to be completed during the communication process so that the desired outcome of communication is achieved.

*Stating a desired objective during communication* allows the communicator to evaluate the outcome of the communication process.

*Using appropriate language while communication* must be well structured and simple so as to not allow misperception of the communicated information.

## COMMUNICATING WITH PATIENTS—THE 5 A'S BEHAVIOUR CHANGE MODEL

### ▌Learning Objective Background

- Mention two models of communication that can facilitate a doctor–patient relationship.
- Outline and comment on the steps of the 5 A's behaviour change model.
- Draw an action plan for the levels of communication in a doctor–patient encounter.

Two well-studied models of communication can facilitate a competent doctor–patient relationship. These models include the 5 A's behaviour change model and the Kalamazoo Consensus Statement (discussed subsequently).

### THE 5 A'S BEHAVIOUR CHANGE MODEL

This model of patient communication is based on providing a patient action plan at each level of the *5 levels of communication*. These levels include:

1. Assessing the patient.
2. Advising the patient.
3. Agreeing with the patient.
4. Assisting the patient.
5. Arranging for the patient.

*A patient action plan* is provided for each level of communication. This includes:

1. Listing specific goals in behavioural terms.
2. Listing barriers and working out strategies to address the barriers.
3. Specifying a follow-up plan.
4. Sharing the plan with the practice team and patient's social support.

A working plan of the 5A's behaviour model in the doctor–patient relationship can be summarized as follows:

1. **Assessing a patient** must take into account the beliefs, behaviour and knowledge of the patient during his/her consultation in the healthcare set-up. Having the patient periodically complete valid health and behaviour surveys during which feedback is provided can facilitate this process. Such surveys must essentially bring out the barriers to the provision of healthcare from a patient's point of view so that the healthcare team can address them appropriately.

2. **Advising the patient** must provide the patient with specific information about the risks his/her health is subject to following the treatment to be provided as well as the benefits of healthcare that he/she will be receiving. An analysis of the patient's behavioural response to the plan of the proposed health management is done and a change in the patient's behaviour is suggested for the successful outcome of the intervention in the patient's health.

3. **Agreeing with the patient** is carried out by collaboratively setting goals based on the patient's interest and confidence in their ability to change the behaviour. Cooperation of the patient's family will facilitate this process.

4. **Assisting the patient** is carried out by identifying personal barriers in the proposed plan of action. Formulating strategies that overcome these barriers and allow the desired outcome of patient care to be achieved follows this. Social and environmental support largely facilitates this level of communication.

5. **Arranging for the patient** refers to plan of patient follow-up following his/her stay in the hospital. Scheduling subsequent doctor–patient interactions using e-mail or phone call reminders for the same facilitates this process. The patients and their families must be appropriately educated on this level of communication.

In conclusion of this summary of the 5 A's behaviour change model of the doctor–patient communication, it must be noted that this model must be implemented in a healthcare set-up following training of its healthcare providers in patient-centred counselling and empowerment.

## COMMUNICATING WITH PATIENTS—THE KALAMAZOO CONSENSUS STATEMENT

### ▮ Learning Objective Background

- Mention two models of communication that can facilitate a doctor–patient relationship.
- Outline and comment on the steps of the Kalamazoo Consensus Statement.
- Assess the outcome of the Kalamazoo Consensus Statement in a doctor–patient relationship.

The Kalamazoo Consensus Statement–1 identifies seven evidence-based 'essential elements,' or tasks of effective physician-patient communication and provides skill competencies for each element. These elements are in turn sub-categorized and assessed in a Likert scale.

The seven elements that facilitate the doctor–patient communication include:

1. Building a relationship.
2. Opening the discussion.
3. Gathering information.
4. Understanding the patient's perspective.
5. Sharing information.
6. Reaching an agreement.
7. Providing closure of the meeting.

These elements of the Kalamazoo Consensus Statement are graded into one of the following ranks of a Likert scale:

- Done well.
- Needs improvement.
- Not done.
- Not applicable.

Following this, the patient's management is appropriately altered to achieve competent healthcare.

### SUB-CATEGORIES OF THE KALAMAZOO ESSENTIAL ELEMENTS

1. **Building a relationship with the patient** is sub-categorized into the following headings.
   a. Greeting and showing interest in the patient as a person.

    b. Using words that show care and concern throughout the interview.

    c. Using tone, pace, eye contact, and posture that show care and concern.

**2. The sub-categories in opening the discussion include:**

    a. Allowing the patient to complete opening statement without interruption.

    b. Asking, "Is there anything else?" to obtain full set of concern.

    c. Explaining and/or negotiating an agenda for the visit.

**3. Gathering information is carried out by:**

    a. Beginning with the patient's story using open-ended questions ("Tell me about ...").

    b. Clarifying details as necessary with more specific or "yes/no" questions.

    c. Summarizing and giving patient opportunity to correct or add information.

    d. Transiting effectively to additional questions.

**4. Understanding the patient's perspective is mediated by:**

    a. Asking about life events, circumstances and other people that might affect health.

    b. Eliciting patient's beliefs, concerns, and expectations about illness and treatment.

    c. Responding explicitly to patient statements about ideas, feelings, and values.

**5. Sharing information is in turn sub-categorized into:**

    a. Assessing the patient's understanding of problem and desire for more information.

    b. Explaining using words that are easy for patient to understand.

    c. Checking for mutual understanding of diagnostic and/or treatment plans.

    d. Asking whether the patient has any questions.

**6. Reaching an agreement of the proposed patient management is carried out using the following sub-categories of communication:**

    a. Including patient in choices and decisions to the extent she/he desires.

   b. Asking about patient's ability to follow diagnostic and/or treatment plans.

   c. Identifying additional resources as appropriate.

7. **Provision of closure of the doctor–patient interaction is carried out by:**

   a. Asking whether the patient has questions, concerns, or other issues.

   b. Summarizing the doctor–patient encounter.

   c. Clarifying follow-up or contact arrangement.

   d. Acknowledging the patient and closing the interview.

*Note:* Each of the sub-categories of the Kalamazoo elements must be graded in the Likert scale.

Having analyzed the elements of the Kalamazoo Consensus Statement, the healthcare team must collaborate and devise further plan of action with regards to the patient's well-being.

## COMMUNICATING WITH PATIENTS—A CASE-BASED STUDY ON HOW DOCTORS MUST NOT COMMUNICATE

"The patient will never care how much you know, until they know how much you care." *(Terry Canale in his American Academy of Orthopedic Surgeons Vice Presidential Address.)*

### Case 1

The scene is set in the consultation room of a general physician in tertiary care hospital. The physician has been delayed and the female patient has been waiting in the common waiting area for over 1 hour. She has consulted the same doctor 4 days ago and was asked to come for a review if symptoms did not subside completely. Now the patient enters the consulting room.

**Doctor:** (In a bored distracted tone while checking his phone for messages) There is no doubt. Your symptoms are due to gallstones, Ms X. Now, we will get an ultrasound and I'll arrange for a consult with one of our general surgeons, okay?

**Patient:** Surgery? But are you sure doctor? I thought it was just indigestion. You see, we're planning this family trip and I'd hate to ruin it for them.

**Doctor:** (While noting down in Ms X's prescription file and simultaneously asking the nurse to fix an urgent appointment with a particular surgeon consulting in the same hospital) Yes, Ms X, I am quite sure now. This is your health we're talking about. And you can take a holiday anytime. So, we'll just arrange that, okay?

**Patient:** But, doctor......?

**Doctor:** Don't worry! I shall see you after admission, okay? Sister, send in the next patient.

This is a classical example of a physician-centred approach that follows the so-called paternalistic model of doctor–patient relationship. The problems in this approach are as follows.

- There was no eye contact between the doctor and the patient.
- The doctor spoke in monotonous tones while multitasking.
- The doctor just informed the patient of the decisions taken regarding her care and proceeded with the plan, taking the patient's consent for granted.
- The patient was not allowed to ask questions and her concerns were not addressed.
- The patient's previous plan of a holiday was just dismissed out of hand as though of no consequence.

The illness experience of the patient in the above scenario was that the doctor:

- Did not have a humane approach.
- Was not empathetic.
- Was disrespectful of the patient's decisions.
- Acted in a high-handed manner as if he knew what was best, without taking the opinions and choices of the patient into consideration.

## Case 2

The scene and background is similar to that of Case 1.

**Doctor:** (Talks in a brisk, no nonsense tone without any pause, has an expressionless face but maintains eye contact.)

Hello, I was held up in ABC Hospital. That's why I am late. Anyway, I'm sure your symptoms are due to gallstones, Ms X. Now, there are several ways in which to handle this. First of all, you can do nothing and you may not have another attack. Secondly, you can try dieting, cut down the fat in your diet to see how that works for you. Otherwise, you can try surgery.

**Patient:** Oh...

**Doctor:** Now, there are two ways. There's laparoscopic surgery and if you have trouble with that, they may just have to open you up. (This is told in a flat, matter of fact, tone.)

**Patient:** Yes but...

**Doctor:** But it's your choice which surgery you'd like to try. Have you thought about a surgeon, you have anyone in mind?

**Patient:** No.

**Doctor:** Well, there are a few that I can recommend or you can ask around. Good. Now, that's done. No doubts, right? Once you have decided, meet me and we shall proceed, okay? Sister, next patient please!

At first glance, the doctor in Case 2 seems to have communicated to the patient better than the doctor in Case 1 but here too, some problems remain. A comparison of the two reveals the following points with regards to the doctor's communication in Case 2.

- The reason for the long waiting time was told but there was no excuse/apology mentioned.

- There was eye contact between the doctor and the patient, which was good.

- The doctor focused on the patient exclusively, i.e. was not distracted or multitasking.

- The brisk no nonsense tone and continuous delivery of information with no pauses intimidated the patient and stopped her from asking any questions. Also, there was little too much information given along with poor phrasing/choice of words. ("If you have trouble with that, they may just have to open you up".) This may be perceived as a threat/a scare tactic by the doctor.

- The doctor did offer choices regarding surgery but the patient's consent for was, again, taken for granted.

- There was no opening at all for the patient to convey her holiday plan.

Hence, the illness experience of the patient in Case 2 was that the doctor was:
- A little arrogant.
- Only interested in doing his job in the shortest possible time (like in the assembly line of a factory).
- Was not at all interested in how she felt emotionally.
- Was not bothered to ask for her choice and opinion regarding treatment options.
- Was vaguely threatening with regards to the surgical procedure did not give any opening for the patient to get her doubts clarified.

## THE DOCTOR–PATIENT COMMUNICATION—THE WAY IT MUST BE

"Medicine is an art whose magic and creative ability have long been recognized as residing in the interpersonal aspects of patient–physician relationship."                                       —*Hall, et al. 1981*

**Activity:** Student role-play.

*Level in the Miller's Pyramid of Learning:* Shows How

Two groups of students (each group consisting of the doctor and patient) are selected for a role-play, the case scenario being similar to that of the above-mentioned cases. The other students observe and correct the deficiencies of the doctor–patient relation ship after the role-play is completed. A teaching faculty who facilitates the appropriate conduct of the doctor–patient relationship mediates this activity.

The following dialogue between the doctor and patient of the case scenario in discussion gives an idea of how the doctor–patient relationship should be. Students participating in the activity can refer to it and develop their own version of the doctor–patient dialogue that can be presented in the role-play.

**Doctor:** (Talks with a smile, in a normal but firm tone, giving adequate pauses, maintains eye contact and has an open body language). Hello, Ms X, I was held up in ABC Hospital. That's why I am late. Hope you have not been waiting too long.

**Patient:** Oh, it's fine Doctor P. I understand.

**Doctor:** Well from what you've told me, I think the problem might be gallstones now. Did you have any worries or concerns about what it might be?

**Patient:** Well, not exactly, I mean I hoped it was just indigestion but gallstones! Doesn't that mean surgery?

**Doctor:** It is most likely so.

**Patient:** You see we're planning a big family trip soon and I'd hate to ruin it for them. Is there anything I could do on a temporary basis at least, like following a prescribed diet?

**Doctor:** Sure, you can cut down on your fat intake since fat can provoke the attacks. At some point, though, they may have to be removed and we don't want it to go over too long before it becomes serious but listen, it's not an emergency now. Maybe we can work around that family vacation. So, tell me, where do you plan on going and for how long?

**Patient:** Oh, it's not a vacation. Our entire extended joint family will be going for 2 weeks to our native village for thanks-giving. We are getting together after 5 years since only now children's vacation and leave for those with careers has coincided.

**Doctor:** That's wonderful then. I understand your situation. Why don't you do something? Give the information about your native place to the staff nurse outside and I shall see if I can recommend a doctor in the vicinity whom you can approach in case of an emergency. Otherwise, after this trip, meet me again and we will go over your options regarding the surgery. Just avoid fried items till then, okay?

**Patient:** Oh, thank you very much Doctor P. I will fix the next appointment right away!

Let's review all the positive aspects of the above communication by the doctor to his patient.

- The doctor spoke in a friendly non-threatening manner with a smile and maintained eye contact.
- There were adequate pauses in the conversation for the patient to interrupt if needed. Also the patient was explicitly asked to voice any worries/concerns.
- The reason for the long waiting time was informed to the patient in a manner that conveyed respect of the patient's time.
- The focus of the doctor was on the patient alone and his active listening of the patient's concerns with the normal range of facial expressions helped convey his empathy.
- The doctor offered options with regards to the treatment, taking the patient's personal requirements into account. Adequate information was provided so that the patient could take an informed decision but there was no overloading.

Hence, the illness experience of the patient in this dialogue was the most satisfactory among all the above-mentioned case scenarios. This covered almost all aspects of AETCOM module 1.4. Case 2 is an example of **patient-centred approach** that follows both the **informative model** and **interpretative model** of doctor–patient relationship.

## Discussion

### What occurs in the physician-centred approach?
- The mind of the doctor focuses on the disease process alone.
- The intention of talking to the patient is only to provide information to the physician so that he can make a diagnosis of

the illness, so that required medical or surgical intervention can be done.

- Here, it is the doctor's experience and interpretation of the patient's illness that is of importance.
- As the physician is thinking in terms of biomedical pathology of the disease, the individual patient context may not be heard.
- An individual patient's experience of and interaction with the disease process is not considered helpful, hence the frequent use of the term 'subjective' for the patient's experience of the illness.

## What occurs in the patient-centred approach?

- The doctor values the individual patient's understanding of the illness as well as the biomedical information needed to manage the disease.
- This contributes to the ability of the doctor to provide high quality care for the patient.
- Patient-centred care has been shown to lead to better outcomes.

Being physician-centred does not mean being a bad physician. Application of biomedical expertise is necessary, but not sufficient in clinical care.

Being patient-centred does not mean complying and giving a patient everything they request. This approach means being respectful of the patient's point of view and arriving at a management plan that is acceptable to both the patient and physician.

A review of research studies conducted over the past two decades have given an overview of the errors in communication made by doctors as under four main themes.

1. Non-verbal communication errors.
2. Verbal communication errors.
3. Errors related to content of information communicated.
4. Errors related to poor attitude of the doctor.

## This can be further understood as follows:

*Errors in non-verbal communication*

- Lack of eye contact through increasingly widespread use of technology.
- Negative facial expressions imply disinterest and lead to feelings of anger and frustration in the patients who feel that personalized care is lacking.

- Non-verbal communication between people based on how the words are said is called paralanguage. These include tone, pitch, pacing, intonation and volume of the voice as well as rhythm and speed of speech. When not used in the right manner, this induces resentment and negativity towards the doctor from the patient's side.
- Body language cues like posture, gesture, facial expression and spatial distance can also convey weariness, disinterest and lack of empathy.

*Errors in verbal communication*

- Lack of active listening by the doctor: This is when the doctor fails to answer the questions of the patient and his attenders but instead proceeds to ask other questions which are important to the doctor from the diagnostic or therapeutic point of view. Also patients felt ignored when they were not given a chance to get their queries cleared or were interrupted when they were putting forth questions to the doctor.
- Inappropriate choice of words: This occurs many a time during night shifts in the hospital or in the casualty/emergency services, when doctors may speak in a brusque, insensitive, threatening and rude manner.

*Content of information communicated*

- The information provided is inadequate: Patients expect the doctors to provide detailed explanation regarding the results of the investigations and the planned management. Doctors are also expected to be 'information engaging'. The lack of regular updates regarding the patient's condition or making arrangements for a patient to undergo surgery (even when there is an absolute indication) without providing all the necessary information and obtaining at least verbal consent—all these are a strict no-no from the patient's point of view.
- The provided information is of poor quality: One of the main reasons of patient's dissatisfaction is that doctors do not clearly explain the rationale behind their recommendations. Sometimes, these may be beyond the purview of the medical personnel such as related to the standard of care based on the available infrastructure, personality of the paramedical staff, etc.

The attitude of the doctor is in turn determined by the above-mentioned characteristics of the doctor–patient encounter.

## RECOMMENDED STUDENT-EXERCISES AND REFLECTION

| Topic | Student-exercise/s | Student-reflection |
|---|---|---|
| Essential principles of communication for the health professional—an overview | • Students must design a role-play amongst them during availaible time and reflect on the landmarks, facilitators and barriers of the communication process | • The students must remember the landmarks of the communication process in healthcare while communicating to health professionals<br>• The students must use facilitators of the communication process to overcome the barriers that may be encountered while communicating during their professional duties |
| Communicating with patients—the 5 A's behaviour change model | • The students must note and discuss the levels of the 5 A's behaviour change model of communication with their facilitator/s during the period of early clinical exposure in phase 1 of their studies | • The students must always reflect on the 5 levels of the 5 A's behaviour change model of communication and draw out a plan for the patient when faced with a doctor–patient interaction |
| Communicating with patient—the Kalamazoo Consensus Statement | • The students must note and discuss the guidelines of the Kalamazoo consensus statement with their facilitator/s during the period of early clinical exposure in phase 1 of their studies | • The students must reflect on the outcome of the doctor–patient relationship if any one of the 7 elements of communication in the Kalamazoo Consensus Statement is *not* adhered to |
| Communicating with patients—a case-based study on how doctors *must not* communicate | • The students must design a case for a role-play amongst them on how communication during the doctor–patient interaction *must not be.* | • The students must reflect on their response as a patient if the doctor that they visit in a hospital *does not* adheres to the essential principles of the communication protocol |

| The doctor–patient communication—the way it *must be* | • The students must design a case for a role-play amongst them on how communication during the doctor–patient interaction *must be*. | • The students must reflect on their response as a patient if the doctor that they visit in a hospital adheres to the essential principles of the communication protocol. |

## SESSION I

### Explorative Session

Large group discussion.

## EXERCISE FOR STUDENTS

**Reflections:** The students should note the key points of the discussion/lecture/microteaching session of principle of communicate.

_____

_____

_____

_____

_____

_____

_____

_____

_____

_____

_____

_____

_____

_____

_____

_____

## SESSION II

### Self-directed Learning (2 hours)

The students should explore the lecture notes and discuss among themselves the methodology of effective communication.

### EXERCISE FOR STUDENTS

**Reflections:** The students should note the gist of their self-directed learning.

_____

_____

_____

_____

_____

_____

_____

_____

_____

_____

_____

_____

_____

_____

_____

_____

_____

_____

_____

_____

_____

## SESSION III

### Small Group Discussion

A 2-hour session for discussion among students regarding the right and wrong methods of doctor–patient communication, how these skills can be modified and best techniques being learnt. The students may enact a role play for the same.

### EXERCISE FOR STUDENTS

**Reflections:** The student may write their observations of the session.

_____

_____

_____

_____

_____

_____

_____

_____

_____

_____

_____

_____

_____

_____

_____

_____

_____

_____

_____

_____

## SESSION IV

Concluding session of discussion and closure of the module (1 hour).

## EXERCISE FOR STUDENTS

The students may present the knowledge and skills gained by them after learning the module. The same may be recorded.

_____

_____

_____

_____

_____

_____

_____

_____

_____

_____

_____

_____

_____

_____

_____

_____

_____

_____

_____

_____

## ASSESSMENT

The formative assessment may be done from their performance in class and the record book.

### Short Answer Questions

1. Define the term 'communication' with regard to a healthcare set-up.

2. What must communication in a healthcare set-up serve to achieve?

3. Outline the landmarks of the communication process.

4. List the types of communication encountered in a medical college/hospital.

5. Mention the barriers that can affect the communication process in a healthcare set-up.

6. Name the factors that can facilitate effective communication in a doctor–patient relationship.

7. What are the 5 A's of the behaviour change model of the doctor–patient relationship?

8. State the action plan that must be used to address the 5 A's of the behaviour change model of the doctor–patient relationship.

9. Mention the seven elements of the Kalamazoo Consensus Statement used to evaluate the doctor–patient relationship.

10. Mention the sub-categories of the seven elements of the Kalamazoo Consensus Statement.

11. What is meant by a doctor-centred approach in healthcare?

12. What is meant by a patient-centred approach in healthcare?

13. Mention the errors of verbal communication in a doctor–patient encounter.

14. Mention the errors of non-verbal communication in a doctor–patient encounter.

15. Mention the errors that allow content of information to be mis-communicated in a doctor–patient encounter.

_____

_____

_____

_____

_____

_____

_____

_____

_____

_____

_____

_____

_____

_____

_____

_____

_____

_____

_____

_____

_____

_____

_____

*The author would like to thank:*

1. *The Medical Education Department of the Christian Medical College—Vellore, for their enrichment on the communication process in healthcare, during the period of the author's training in the Revised Basic Course Workshop and Advanced Course in Medical Education.*

2. *Dr C Anithu, Assistant Professor, Department of Physiology, Chettinad Hospital and Research Institute, for her input into structuring the article so as to suit the first phase medical student's understanding of the same.*

# Cadaver as Our First Teacher

*Krishna Garg*

## HISTORY OF CADAVERIC DISSECTION

Physicians of ancient Greece gained information about health and human body. The information ended with Hippocrates who laid the foundation of a medical school in the island of Cos in the fifth century BC.

Herophilus, disciple of Hippocrates from Cos became a very much respected anatomist in the school of Alexandria. Herophilus is known as father of scientific anatomy.

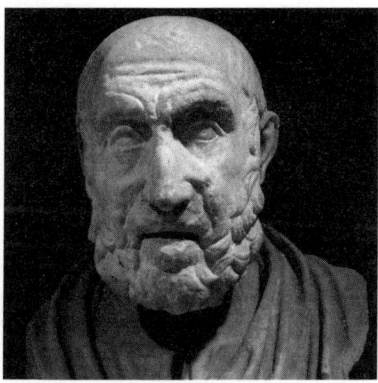

Hippocrates

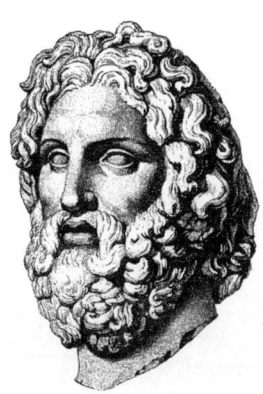

Herophilus

Anatomical dissection was done in a systemic way in Alexandria. But another disciple of Herophilus, Filinns, from Cos argued that dissection has no practical utility.

Galen from Greece introduced Greek Medicine and became a successful physician in Rome. He wrote 'Treaty of Anatomy', which was used for teaching for more than 14 centuries till the Middle Ages. In Europe during the Middle Ages (till 13th century), dissection was prohibited. Anatomy was taught by Galen's texts.

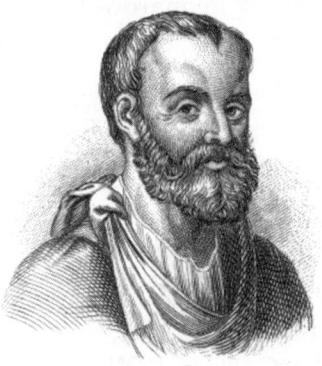

Galen

During 14th and 15th centuries some professors of Italian and French Universities started using cadavers as teaching tools. Mordinodei Luzzi (1275–1326) introduced dissection again by doing public dissections. He published a manual Anatomia (De anatome) which was the textbook for next 3 centuries in future. Andreas Versalius from University of Pradua published

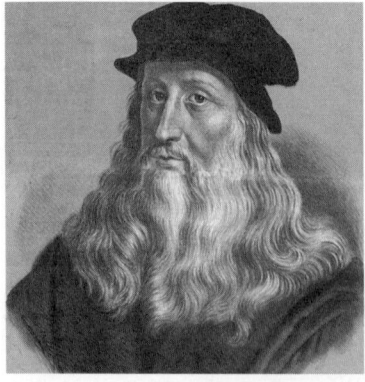

Leonardo-da-Vinci

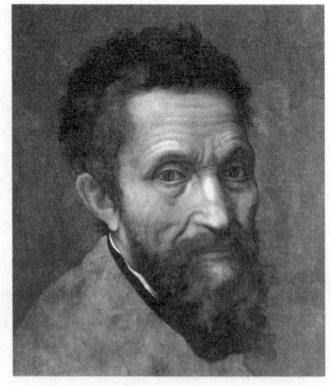

Michelangelo

De humanicorporisfabrica (1543)—a masterpiece manual. According to him cadavers were considered like 'books'. The interest in dissections and skeleton increased. Jacob Berengario da Capri named the skeletal parts.

Alessandro Achillini wrote Carports humanianatomica and Anatomicae annotations described 7 tarsal bones.

Artwork by painters, e.g. Leonardo-da-Vinci 1452–1519 and Michelangelo helped in learning anatomy. They illustrated the body in its natural splendour. Leonardo-da-Vinci developed cross sectional anatomy.

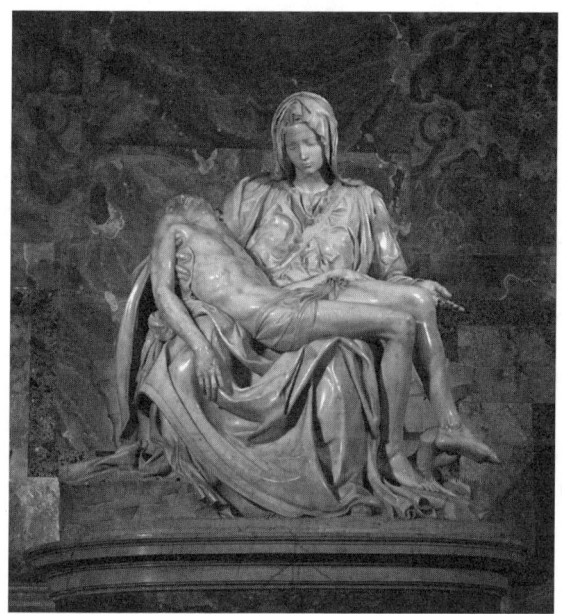

Art work by Michelangelo

Marcello Malpighi developed histology in 17th century. During 18th century interest developed in embryology.

Honere Fragonard made his anatomical specimens into art peices. His works are on display near Paris, France.

First Medical School in America was founded in 1765 at College of Philadelphia. During 19th century demand for cadavers increased. Cadavers legally available were those of executed criminals. Robbing of graves was seen in and people were punished. In New York a doctor was dissecting a female body. The doctor waved to a boy through a window showing 'hand', he was dissecting. The boy recognised the hand belonging to his mother who had died recently.

In Edinburg, Scotland, William Burke and William Hare used to intoxicate guests with alcohol, murder them by intoxication and then sell their bodies. They were found guilty of murdering 16 people. Bruke was hung, dissected and exhibited (Tward and Patterson 2002).

In 1831, Massachusetts' Anatomical Act was passed which established that only unclaimed bodies can be used for anatomical dissection (Dyer and Thorndike 2000).

During 1968 Unifor Anatomy Gift Act was adopted, where voluntary donations of dead body was accepted (Jones 1991).

Plastination technique created by Mr Gunther Von Hagenes at Heidelberg University in Germany (Weiglein 1977) is used in teaching and research. The exhibition of plastinated specimens is called 'Body World' and is extremely good and knowledgeable. Mr Gunther is known as 'Mr Death'. While on a trip to New York, I happened to see an 'ad' of 'Body Worlds'. I requested my son to take me to this exhibition. He left his friends for shopping and took me to this 'awesome art work of Body Worlds'. This made my trip an unforgettable one.

**Mexico:** At present anatomy is taught by dissection in addition to bones, models and multimedia programmes. USA and Canada maintain that dissection will be supplemented by multimedia learning.

**India:** During 2nd and 3rd century, Arthashastra described four ways of dying, e.g. drowning, hanging, strangulating and asphyxiation. Practice of dissection was followed during 7th and 8th centuries. It was rightly felt that better understanding of anatomy would create better surgeons. Female doctors were also trained in India well before those in England.

Anatomical teachings including dissection from India spread throughout the world. But the practice of dissection was stunted by Islam.

In 1827, a student **Pandit Madusudan Gupta** performed good human dissections. He joined the newly created Ayurvedic classes in Sanskrit College in Calcutta in 1826. He was promoted to the post of a teacher in the same medical college in view of his great interest and enthusiasm. He was the first man who dissected a cadaver in 1836 and created a sensation in orthodox Hindu society. He was honored by a 7 cannon salute.

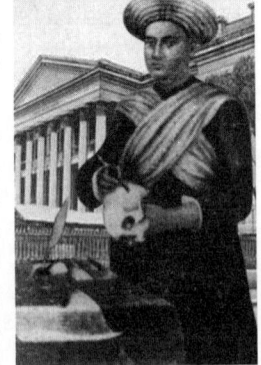

Pandit Madusudan Gupta

## Method of Dissection during Ayurvedic Period

That is dead body of a man, having all its parts, not dead by either poison or long standing (chronic) disease, not of hundered years of age should be obtained; feces present in the intestines should be removed; then the body is wrapped either with manja grass, valkala (inner bark of trees), kusa grass, sana (hemp) or any such material, tied well and placed inside a cage, which is kept in a slow running stream, at a hidden place and allowed to undergo putrification. After knowing that it has become properly putrified, it should be taken out, removed of its binding and investigated for 7 days, scrubbing it slowly (carefully) with brushes made from usira grass, vala (hairs of tail of animals), venu (bamboo), balvaja (a kind of grass) or any other similar material and observe with his own eyes, all the major and minor parts like the skin, etc. described earlier. (Shushruta Sharir 5/49).

The current state of dissection is bad. The number of cadavers are few despite the enormous population. The number of months for first professional has been decreasing. It was 2 years till about 1970, when it got reduced to 1½ years. As of now since 2000 it is further reduced to one year. For a first year student, it takes 1–2 months to get used to the hostel. They feel lots of 'home sickness'. The course is taught 'fast' because of paucity of time. Students take time to understand the 'infamous difficult to master subject'. Their basic knowledge remains 'poor'.

**Islamic World:** Islamic faith was applied in Islamic world. Islamic laws have discouraged us from practice of dissection-commented by Ibn-al-Nasif a physician and Muslim jurist. Prior to 10th century, dissection was not done on human cadavers. After 12th century dissection was forbidden.

In 1952, Islamic School of Jurisprudence in Egypt allowed autopsy. It is permitted for medical and judicial purposes. Human dissection is present in modern day Islamic World, but is not published due to social stigma.

**Tibet:** These people had long experience in anatomy. Tibetans adopted 'sky burial'—starts with ritual dissection of the deceased, followed by feeding parts to vultures. Tibetan anatomical knowledge was mentioned in Ayurveda and also in Chinese medicine.

Christian Europe—dissection was rare during Middle Ages but it was practised during 13th century and they thought that human cadaver was no longer seen as sacrosanct. Middle Ages saw the revival of interest in medical studies, dissection and autopsy.

Mondino de Luzzi carried out first recorded public dissection around 1315. Galeazzo di Santa Sofia made first public dissection in Vienna in 1404.

Versalius in 16th century carried out numerous dissections. He lectured and dissected simultaneously.

In modern Europe dissection is practised in biological research and education.

Britain: In 16th century limited rights were given to physicians and surgeons to dissect cadavers.

Mid-18th century Royal College of Physicians and Company of Barber-Surgeons were permitted to do dissections.

Murder Act 1752 allowed bodies of executed murderess to be dissected for anatomy.

19th century-infamous Burke and Hare murders in 1828 where 16 people murdered to be sold to anatomists.

Anatomy Act 1832—increased legal supply of cadavers for dissection. Peninsula College of Medicine and Dentistry UK founded in 2000, became first Modern Medical School to carry out anatomy education without dissection.

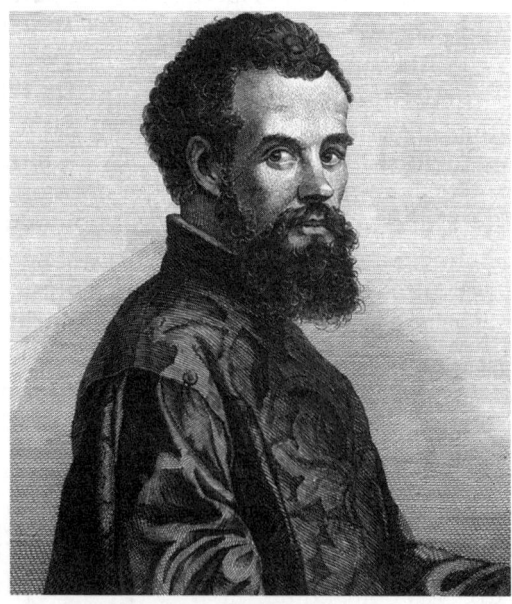

Versalius

Traditional dissection is supported by many teachers and students. They say "using a scalpel on an actual recently living person is an entirely different matter as compared to colorful chart of anatomy".

## Cadaver as a First Teacher

Once a senior secondary school student with biology gets admission in a medical college. She is renamed as a medical student, who is mentally prepared to study for about 10 years before becoming a specialized doctor. During the first professional period a medical student needs to study anatomy, physiology and biochemistry.

From time immemorial, anatomy has been viewed as a complex and challenging subject to be learnt from embalmed human cadaver who is slowly and steadily being dissected. As one does dissection in a group, one is incorporating a great skill including the teamwork and patience. So, globally it is acclaimed that the cadaver is the First Teacher.

## How to Obtain a Cadaver

Cadaver is a dead human body used in scientific or medical research.

Earlier and even at present, unclaimed dead bodies usually belonging to poor strata are taken by the police. Police personnel inform the medical college (anatomy department) to collect the body. Even if postmortem has been done, the body is taken by the anatomy department for the dissection of the limbs. For the last decade or so many persons make a 'Will' to donate their bodies. To promote this scheme, many anatomy departments give it as a news item in the local newspapers. The department puts the photograph of the voluntary donor outside the Dissection Hall.

## Preservation of the Cadavers

The dead body starts putrifying and decaying within few hours after death depending on the weather. To prevent this, bodies are embalmed with formalin mixture. Procedure of embalming takes few hours to complete.

Embalming is also done if a dead body or cadaver is to be transported to a distant place in the country or abroad. Even if a VIPs body is to be kept for public viewing before the last rites the body has to be embalmed. Embalming can be done as: (i) arterial embalming, (ii) cavity embalming, (iii) hypodermic embalming and (iv) surface embalming.

Embalming fluid—the fluid is prepared by thoroughly mixing up 5 litres of water 3 litres of formalin (40%), 2 litres of spirit, 1 litre of glycerine, sodium chloride, etc.

The cadaver is put in a supine position on a table. It is shaved and cleaned.

**Procedure for arterial embalming:** A 6 cm long vertical incision is given in the upper medial side of thigh. After reflecting skin and fasciae, femoral sheath is incised to visualise the femoral artery. The prepared embalming fluid is put in the embalming machine which is connected to a cannula.

A small nick is given in the femoral artery and cannula introduced so that its tip points towards the head end and 8.5 litres of fluid is pumped under 20 pounds pressure. Then the direction of cannula is reversed and rest of the fluid is pumped in. Lastly, the skin and fasciae are stitched.

**Cavity embalming:** The internal fluids inside the body cavities are replaced with embalming chemicals with the use of an aspirator and trochar.

**Hypodermic embalming:** Injection of embalming fluid into tissues with the help of a syringe and needle. It is done in an area where arterial fluid has not reached.

**Surface embalming:** Preserves areas on skin damaged by accidents or skin donations.

## Embalming and Ethics

The decision for embalming is taken by close relatives usually when there is a 'Will' to the same effect. This trend is 'catching up' and some people are 'making a Will' to donate their body for education or research to the department of anatomy. Earlier and even now many bodies are the 'unclaimed ones'.

**Care of the cadaver:** The cadaver has to be handled with care and respect. Only the part being dissected is kept open and exposed, rest is to be covered by a sheet. After dissection the dissecting part must also be covered palms and soles are wrapped till their dissection is reached. Over the weekend or a holiday the cadaver or the body is put in a formalin tank to be taken out after the weekend. There is always an irritating smell of formalin causing watering of the eyes but it gets over within 30–40 minutes. Detached limbs are to be wrapped up by a bandage to prevent drying. If fungus is seen on a part, it must be removed by using dilute carbolic acid. "You care for the cadaver, he or she takes care of your learning anatomy".

So, a cadaver, a dead human body is showing his internal features to help you learn anatomy and Cadaver is the First Teacher. The students of University of Taiwan are told about the family of the cadaver. They visit the family to pay their respects as their deceased family member is assisting them to become a doctor for treating the patients.

Many institutions start their anatomy dissection classes with a prayer to thank Almighty for giving them a body to learn. At a college in Mumbai, the cadaveric oath is administered to first year medical undergraduates who pledge to honour the dignity and integrity of the human remains that they are about to work on. Anatomical memorial services are held in Mayo Medical College, Rochester, USA, to enable students to reflect on the life of the departed souls who facilitated their education. The cadaver in addition to teaching anatomy also teaches to work in a team. Even after many years of dissection one remembers colleagues of your dissection table and the happy hours spent together. We must all remember that the cadaver was one of us and deserve great respect. Cadaver not only teaches gross anatomy also surface anatomy and embryology from dissection of the fetuses.

**Disposal of the cadaver:** The remains of the cadaver are buried in the burial ground attached to the department of anatomy.

The cadaver continues to be a teacher in Forensic Medicine. Here the cause of death has to be established by postmortem so that guilty persons may be punished.

**Present scenario:** As early as 1956, two students got a limb for dissection. Most of the students enjoyed the dissection periods. Gradually the ratio of number of cadavers versus the number of students decreased. Many more students were allotted a limb. Then two students of a group were allotted a day for dissection to provide them a feeling of a young surgeon. Slowly and steadily the availability of the cadavers further reduced and students gradually lost interest in the dissection. This was further compounded by the fact that time allotted for first professional course decreased from 2 years to 1½ year and then to 1 year. Thus the time became too little during which the whole course has to be learnt, understood and recapitulated. The feel of real dissection remains within ones fingers and brain and can never be compensated by virtual imaging.

As the dissection continues one starts to recognise the cadaver, develops respect for the cadaver. Along with the dissection students have to study the bones. The bones have to be purchased as a set of bones. As of now many students do not even buy the bone set. The real bones over a period of time have became too expensive and the synthetic bones hardly reveal any features. Thus the students do not dissect as the cadavers are not available; do not study from bones as they do not possess a bone set; do not practise drawing of colored diagrams for reasons best known to them; their knowledge is poor.

**To me as a teacher of anatomy:** Anatomy is action. Try and dissect, study from the bones, do movements on your own body feel the contracting muscles; draw colored diagrams; mark the arteries, veins, nerves, etc. on your own body and one will not forget anatomy.

**Computers potential for teaching anatomy:** In 1988 the Visible Human Project of US National Library of Medicine began. Now anatomy is being integrated with radiographs. CT, MRI, sectional anatomy scans to provide a 3D view of anatomy. The alternatives to dissection are computer programmes, videos, etc. being developed with the help of computers. This method is as dynamic as a cinema.

| Human cadaveric dissection | Alternative to dissection/artificial cadaver synthetic corpse |
| --- | --- |
| Preservation required | No preservation required |
| More staff required for maintenance | Less staff required for maintenance |
| Trained staff can manage | Highly trained staff can manage to teach |
| Scalpels, etc. required | Scalpels, etc. not required |
| Cannot be used repeatedly | Can be used repeatedly |
| Actual feel of a nerve, artery is there | Actual feel of nerve, artery, muscle is not there |

**Ideal method** is dissection with added technology.

**Dress code for the students:** The students must wear an apron or overall, a cap, gloves to protect from any injury, etc.

## DISSECTION INSTRUMENTS

Large instruments like hammer, saw, chisel, etc. are provided in the department. Every medical student must have the following instruments in his/her dissection box.

**Scalpel:** The scalpel is used for giving incisions. It should have a detachable blade of 3–4 cm. Scalpel blade should be sharp and scalpel handle need to be metallic. Care must be taken not to injure oneself.

**Forceps:** Forceps are used to hold the part being dissected. One pair should be serrated tip forceps for lifting the nerve, artery or vein, etc. Another pair should be toothed forceps for holding the structure firmly while dissection is being done. Size of the forceps may be 7.5 cm to 15 cm.

**Scissors:** Pair of small scissors is necessary for cutting a small structure. Another pair of big scissors (15 cm) is also required at times.

**Probe:** The probe is useful for doing blunt dissection and for cleaning the dissecting region.

**Hand lens:** The handlens is required to magnify the smaller structures for better and correct identification.

## DISSECTION TECHNIQUE

Mark the lines of incision with a chalk.

**Removal of the skin:** First a small incision is given in the skin. The edge of skin is firmly grasped by the toothed forceps and separated from the underlying superficial fascia with the help of the scalpel. The skin thus separated is reflected on one side. It is still attached to part of the body. The superficial fascia contains cutaneous nerves, veins, and arteries. After the study of these structures this fascia and fat is removed and the deep fascia is exposed.

Deep fascia is dense and tough. It needs to be removed to see the deeper muscles, main arteries veins, nerves and lymph nodes, etc. One has to follow 'steps of dissection' from the dissector or textbook.

Dissection is done regionwise—upperlimb, thorax, lower limb, abdomen and pelvis, head and neck, brain. The order followed may be different in various institutions.

## EXERCISE FOR STUDENTS

### SESSION I

### Exploratory Session (2 hours)

Arrange an explorative lecture session addressing the students about the advantages of dissecting a cadaver, procedure of procuring and looking after it during the dissection hours and after the dissection hours and disposal of the dissected cadaver followed by a group discussion.

**Reflections:** The students should note the key points of the lecture and summaries the knowledge gained by them.

_____

_____

_____

_____

_____

_____

_____

_____

_____

_____

_____

_____

_____

_____

_____

_____

_____

_____

_____

_____

_____

## SESSION II

The students should present in small group regarding the learnt topic in the form of presentation, poster, sketches, elocution, etc.

**Reflections:** The students should record the observations of activities carried out by them.

_____

_____

_____

_____

_____

_____

_____

_____

_____

_____

_____

_____

_____

_____

_____

_____

_____

_____

_____

_____

_____

_____

_____

_____

_____

## ANATOMY ACT

**Anatomy Act** is an act promoted by Legislature and published in the Gazette. The Act regulates the use of dead bodies for medical purposes. Anatomy Act was enacted in India in 1948. The Anatomy Act provides for the supply of unclaimed bodies of deceased persons to medical institution for the purpose of medical education/research by means of dissection. 'Anatomy' means study of human body; 'teacher of medicine'—person who is engaged or employed as a teacher of anatomy in an authorized institution established under this Act.

Ministry of health authorizes establishment of colleges where study of anatomy is carried out.

The college has to be granted a license to practice anatomy. Duly licensed colleges can receive the dead body for dissection. Only colleges/institutions having lawful custody of bodies may permit anatomical dissection.

If a person, either in writing at any time during his/her life or verbally in the presence of two or more witnesses during the illness directs that his/her body by given to a medical/ dental college after death; then the body may be sent in a coffin to the authorized college. The dead body has to be kept for a period of 48 hours before it is sent to the college for dissection/ research—for the relatives to take back the body. Even if the dead body/cadaver has been embalmed, the relatives staying far away can claim the body from the college under supervision of the police.

The dissection has to be done in a quiet and decent manner. The parts of the body have to buried/cremated after dissection. Anatomy Act does not prohibit postmortem examination. Such bodies can also be used for dissection/research. Any person who contravenes the provisions of this Act shall be guilty of an offence and is liable for a fine or imprisonment as decided by the state.

Since the demand for bodies is gradually increasing, persons have been coming forward to donate their bodies. There have been awareness camps to this effect and many people have registered for body donation, with or without filling the requisite form.

So, Anatomy Act helps in ideal learning of anatomy, which prepares him/her to be a better physician/surgeon.

## The Following Poem 'Thus Spoke the Cadaver' Explains his Emotional Aspects

Handle me with little love and care
As I had missed it in my life affair
Was too poor for cremation or burial
That is why am lying in dissection hall

You dissect me, cut me, section me
But your learning anatomy should be precise
Worry not, you would not be taken to court
As I am happy to be with the bright lot

Couldn't dream of a fridge for cold water
Now my body parts are kept in refrigerator
Young student sit around me with friends
Few dissect, rest talk, about food, family and movies
How I enjoy the dissection periods
Don't you? Unless you are interrogated by a teacher

When my parts are buried post dissection
Bones are taken out for the skeleton
Skeleton is the crown glory of the museum
Now I am being looked up by great enthusiasm

If not as skeletons as loose bones
I am in their bags and in their hostel rooms
At times, I am on their beds as well

Oh, what promotion to heaven from hell
I won't leave you, even if you pass anatomy
Would follow you in forensic medicine and pathology
Would be with you even in clinical teaching
Medicine line is one where dead teach the living

One humble request I'd make
Be sympathetic to persons with disease
Don't panic, you'll have enough money
And I bet, you'd be singularly happy.

## Short Answer Questions

1. Who were the first physicians to gain information about human body?

2. Who founded the first medical school? Who is known as Father of Scientific Anatomy?

3. Who wrote 'Treaty of Anatomy'?

4. Which manual was published by Andreas Versalius?

5. Name the scientists who did artwork on anatomy?

6. Where and when was the first medical school founded?

7. How were the cadavers for dissection provided?

8. What did Burke and Hare do to provide cadavers in Edinburg, Scotland?

9. In which year was Massachusetts' Anatomical Act passed?

10. Who started the Plastination technique of embalming the bodies?

11. Name the four ways of dying as described in Arthshastra?

12. Name the Indian who performed good human dissections?

13. Why is cadaver called First Teacher?

14. How are the cadavers obtained for dissection purposes?

15. What are the methods used to preserve the cadavers?

16. How is the care of the cadaver taken?

17. How is the cadaver after dissection disposed?

18. What are the alternatives to human dissection?

19. What is the dress code for the medical students?

20. Name the instruments which first year medical students must possess.

21. Can the cadaver be the first patient also?

22. Give points in favour and against the dissection versus multimedia learning.

23. Make a small poem in favour of learning anatomy.

24. Suggest few new methods of learning anatomy.

# Appendix 1

# History of Medicine

*Suyog Sindhu*

## ▌ Medicine in Early Civilizations

Medicine developed at an early stage in **Egypt, India** and **China**. The earliest Indian and Chinese medical texts that we possess are decidedly younger than those of Egypt. While Egyptian medicine completed its course long ago, ancient Indian and Chinese medicine are still fully alive and are practiced by millions of people even today.

## EGYPT

The medicine of ancient Egypt shaped ideas of the civilizations around it, including the medicine of Greek and Roman civilizations. Ancient Egyptians had a widespread reputation for their medical knowledge. Each of the physicians of Egypt was a specialist committed to one particular branch of medicine. The foundation of medical science was established in Egypt more than fifty centuries ago as evidenced by a mass of documentary evidence, medical 'Papyri'. According to the Kahun papyri, it was determined whether a woman would or would not be able to bear children by keeping a bulb of onion or garlic in her vagina over night until dawn. If the specific odor of either appeared in her mouth, she would be able to bear children. The scientific foundation of this fertility test is that onion and garlic contain volatile oils which pass from the cervix through the uterus to the fallopian tubes and, if these are unobstructed, reach the peritoneal cavity which has a very high absorbency to circulation. The route of excretion of these volatile oils is the respiratory tract. The first specialized hospitals for antenatal care were established in Egypt 4000 years ago. A separate room called *Mameze* was built in the house garden or upper story to isolate the mother for 2 weeks after giving birth and to protect her from puerperal sepsis.

The ancient Egyptians practiced family planning. For example, contraceptive devices of different shapes and sizes were inserted into the uterus. They believed that semen was formed in a man's heart and stored in the holy bone called the sacrum. Topical anesthesia was necessarily practised for minor operations. By putting vinegar (acetic acid) in a certain concentration over marble stone, a cooling effect of carbon dioxide resulted from the interaction with acetic acid. The marble stone thus had an anesthetizing effect!

Trephining, the process of perforating the skull with a surgical instrument was common surgical practice. Skulls of mummies with well-healed edges indicate that patients lived after a trephine operation.

The ancient Egyptians practiced venesection or bloodletting. Earlier as well as today physicians use this procedure to treat scorpion stings or snakebites.

Egyptian orthopedicians used wooden splints padded with linen and *imru*, which seems to resemble plaster of Paris.

One of the techniques mentions soaking linen with egg white, wrapping it around the fractured limb after its reduction, and then leaving it to dry.

There were superb techniques in the field of dentistry as well. They used the cavity of a recently extracted tooth or prepared a cavity in the jawbone, then placed a healthy tooth inside the cavity and fixed it to an adjacent tooth using a fine gold wire. They had learnt that the transplant was not rejected if the tooth came from a twin but might be rejected if the tooth came from a person unrelated to the family of the patient.

## CHINA

Traditional Chinese Medicine (TCM) is an integral part of ancient Chinese civilization. Diagnosis is based on observing, listening or smelling, questioning, touching, knowing the family, family history and food likes-dislikes. Treatment is based on knowledge acquired through long-term medical practice in combination with an assessment of natural conditions including climate, geography and phenology (the study of periodic effects on plant and animal life cycles influenced by seasonal variations).

There is also an ancient tradition for herbal medicine in China.

In prehistoric times, people ate plants, fruits from trees and grasses, worms, and clams (a marine bivalve mollusc with shells of equal size). Later on herbs with medicinal values were discovered and used for treating diseases.

Archeological investigations have found inscriptions and characters on bones and tortoise shells dealing with diseases like headache, abdominal pain, dizziness, common cold, tinnitus, deafness, eye disease, and ulcers, as well as children's and women's diseases and dental diseases such as caries. They also included infectious diseases and parasitosis.

In one of the Chinese medical literature it is mentioned— "diseases can be seen in all seasons, e.g. head disease in spring, scabies and other itching diseases in summer, malaria and cold diseases in autumn, and asthmatic and coughing diseases in winter"—this indicates the recognition of relationships between seasons and diseases by ancient Chinese.

## INDIA

Archeological and modern genetic evidences suggest that human populations have migrated into the Indian subcontinent since prehistoric times. The knowledge of the medicinal value of plants and other substances and their uses go back to the time of the earliest settlers. Excavations at different sites suggest that medical interventions such as dentistry and trepanation were practiced as early as 7000 BCE in the Indian subcontinent.

**Ayurveda** is the indigenious system of medicine that developed here over a span of several ages. In Sanskrit it means 'science or wisdom (*veda*) of life'. It is a rationale, logical medical science which has survived from antiquity to the present day. Historical roots suggest that it has paved the way for various branches of medicine.

There is collection of anatomical data from ancient India. During the practice of Vedic sacrifice, the anatomy of the sacrificised animal was carefully studied. A crude form of the human body dissection to acquire anatomical knowledge was probably practiced in early times but later the study of anatomy became less important for pattern of medicine followed here.

The idea central to Ayurveda is that 'five great elements'—earth, water, fire, air and space—make up the entire phenomenal world including the human body. Further a whole system of dietary recommendations forms framework for diagnosis, therapy and treatment in this traditional medicine. It comprises recommendations ranging from preparation and consumption of food, to healthy routines for day and night, sexual life, and rules for ethical conduct. For example, in dietetics it is considered that sweet foods are predominantly made up of the elements—earth and water. In the human body fatty tissue is made up mainly of the same elements. This implies that excessive eating of sweet substances increases fatty tissue in the body, this principle goes hand-in-hand with modern system of medicine! In Ayurvedic practice, the elementary composition of a substance is known by its properties or qualities. The principle is to treat with opposite qualities.

Three ancient books known as the Great Trilogy—'**Charaka Samhita'**, '**Sushruta Samhita**' and '**Astanga Hridaya**' written in Sanskrit more than 2,000 years ago, are considered the main texts on Ayurvedic medicine. The earliest codified documents are **Charaka Samhita** and **Sushruta Samhita**. Charak Samhita deals with internal medicine whereas Sushruta Samhita is dominated by surgical procedures. Sushruta Samhita discusses nine branches—surgery, ear, nose and throat diseases, toxicology, psychiatry, pediatrics, gynecology, sexology, and virility. It relies on a natural and holistic approach to physical and mental health focusing on interconnections among people, their health, the universe, the body's constitution and life forces. Using these concepts, Ayurvedic physicians prescribe individualized treatments that include herbs, diet, music, massage treatments, exercise and meditation along with lifestyle recommendations.

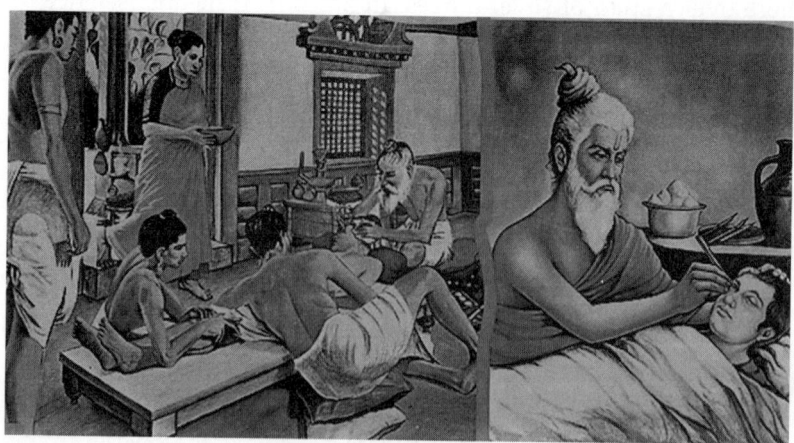

Cataract surgery by Sushruta

This traditional Indian medicine identified a wide range ailments including fever, cough, constipation, diarrhea, dropsy, abscesses, seizures, tumours, and leprosy. Treatments included plastic surgery, lithotomy, tonsillectomy, couching (a form of cataract surgery), puncturing to release fluids in the abdomen, extraction of foreign bodies, treatment of anal fistulas, treating fractures, amputations, cesarean sections and stitching of wounds. The use of herbs and surgical instruments was widespread. Treatments were also prescribed for complex ailments, including angina pectoris, diabetes, hypertension, and stones.

This Indian system of indigenous medicine has regained its importance in present times not only in its country of origin but worldwide!

## TIMELINES IN HISTORY OF MEDICINE

The history of medicine is long and distinguished one as healers sought to alleviate illness and fix injuries since the dawn of human civilization. It is difficult to spot the starting point of this long journey. The finish point is all the more beyond imagination. As it would be an uphill task to dive into the ocean of history and fish out every stepping stone in path of healing, an attempt has been made in this book to highlight the most remarkable discoveries and discoverers in different timelines of history.

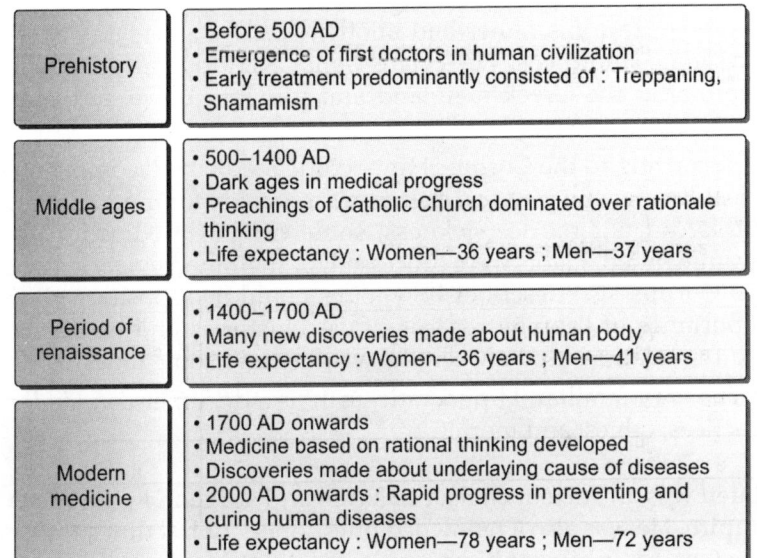

| Prehistory | • Before 500 AD<br>• Emergence of first doctors in human civilization<br>• Early treatment predominantly consisted of : Treppaning, Shamamism |
|---|---|
| Middle ages | • 500–1400 AD<br>• Dark ages in medical progress<br>• Preachings of Catholic Church dominated over rationale thinking<br>• Life expectancy : Women—36 years ; Men—37 years |
| Period of renaissance | • 1400–1700 AD<br>• Many new discoveries made about human body<br>• Life expectancy : Women—36 years ; Men—41 years |
| Modern medicine | • 1700 AD onwards<br>• Medicine based on rational thinking developed<br>• Discoveries made about underlaying cause of diseases<br>• 2000 AD onwards : Rapid progress in preventing and curing human diseases<br>• Life expectancy : Women—78 years ; Men—72 years |

Though there are no fixed points where time can be labelled, history of medicine can be divided in following four timelines in accordance to its advancement.

I. Prehistoric medicine.

II. Middle ages.

III. Period of renaissance.

IV. Modern medicine.

## PROMINENT PHYSICIANS IN PREHISTORIC ERA

**Hippocrates** was born on the Aegean island of Kos around **460 BC**. Little is known about his life experiences. Historians rely on a biography written some 500 years after his death by another Greek physician, Soranus and a collection of medical writings in form of more than 60 medical books commonly called the Hippocratic Corpus.

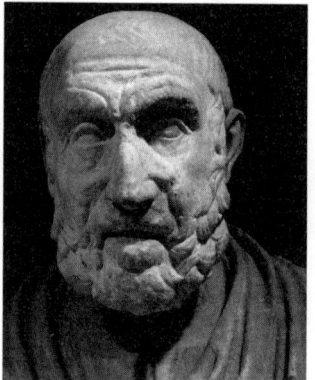

Hippocrates

His formal name was Hippocrates Asclepiades, meaning 'descendant of (the doctor-god) Asclepios'. He was born in a wealthy family, as son of Praxithea and Heracleides. He learnt medicine from his father and another physician Herodicos. Historians believe Hippocrates travelled throughout the Greek mainland and possibly Libya and Egypt practicing medicine.

According to the Corpus, Hippocratic medicine recommended a healthy diet and physical exercise as a remedy for most ailments. If this did not reduce sickness, some type of medication was recommended. Plants were processed for their medicinal elements. The Corpus also describes how joints could be repositioned, the importance of keeping records of case histories and treatments, and the relationship between the weather and some illnesses.

The very familiar 'Hippocratic Oath' is a document on medical practices, ethics, and morals.

**Galen** was an ancient Greek physician and surgeon in the Roman Empire. He was also a renowned philosopher of his times though most of his philosophical writings have been lost. As a very prominent physician, he greatly influenced the development of various scientific disciplines like anatomy, physiology, pathology and neurology, and was considered an authority on medical theory and practice in Europe until the mid-17th century. He was a skilled surgeon and much ahead of his times. He was known to have performed complicated surgeries on delicate organs like eyes and brains. His works on the circulatory system were also much ahead of his times. Galen was a

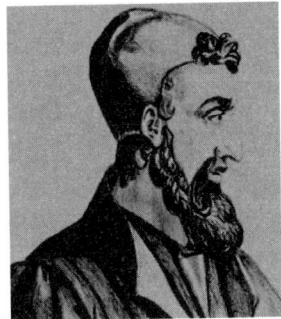

Galen

prolific writer and is believed to have produced more work than any author in antiquity. It is possible that he might have written up to 600 manuscripts. A major fire destroyed most of his works and less than a third of his works have survived. Although he was more famous as a medical practitioner, Galen was also a renowned philosopher of his times. He wrote extensively about logic and philosophy, and integrated philosophical thought with medical practice. His writings were influenced by earlier Greek and Roman thinkers, including Plato, Aristotle, and the Stoics.

## MIDDLE AGES (500-1400 AD)

Doctors in the Middle Ages knew little of the origination for the ailments that they were trying to treat, and not knowing the cause of the ailment made it incredibly difficult to try and figure out a way to treat or prevent it. Most doctors came from the higher end of the social ladder, and were generally more educated. Since the lower class consisted mostly of farmers or servants, their education level was extremely limited. The small amount of information that was available about the medical field made it impossible for doctors in the Middle Ages to properly practice medicine. There was almost no literature available and the literature that could be found was often written in a language that would need to be translated. The fact that the literature was being translated left a large margin of error. People did not travel or learn from other cultures the way that we do today, and that lack of knowledge led to the detriment of the medical field.

Many of the medical practices that existed during this period are no longer used today. Since there was little research done on the human body almost all physicians relied on the literature that was developed by Galen's observations of the human anatomy.

This meant that there were many beliefs that were not accurate. Doctors in the Middle Ages had no way of knowing if it was their practices of the disease itself that was hurting the patient!

Successful cures in that era were what today seem to be crazy cures. For example:

- Bleeding, applying leeches, smelling strong posies or causing purging or vomiting
- Cutting open buboes, draining the pus and making the patient hot or cold, e.g. by taking hot baths
- Trepanning—cutting a hole in the skull
- Praying, or whipping themselves to try to earn God's forgiveness
- Lighting fires in rooms and spreading the smoke, tidying rubbish from the streets and banning new visitors to towns and villages

The practice of medicine in the Middle Ages was rooted in the Greek tradition.

Some of the most notorious illnesses of the Middle Ages were the **plague (the Black Death), leprosy,** and **Saint Anthony's fire. Leprosy** was very disfiguring and therefore sufferers were feared and kept apart. Lepers were obliged to live outside a town or village and to carry a bell to warn people of their approach.

## PERIOD OF RENAISSANCE (1400–1700 AD)

Renaissance medicine is the term used for the development of medicine at the time of the Renaissance in Europe. The renaissance period started in northern Italy during the 14th century and spread to Europe in the late 15th century. It starts from the date of discovery of America by Columbus.

The main change in Renaissance medicine was largely due to the increase in anatomical knowledge, aided by an easing of the legal and cultural restrictions on dissecting cadavers. This allowed doctors to gain a much better understanding of the human body and get rid of techniques that harmed rather than cured.

The surgeons of this era were also categorized as a class system. They were acknowledged as master surgeons, 'surgeons of the long robe,' or the lower class of barber surgeons, 'surgeons of the short robe'!

Discoveries during the Renaissance laid the foundations for a change in thinking leading to the view that the body is made up of specialized systems that work together—the basis of medical knowledge that we still see today.

# IMPORTANT PERSONALITIES IN THE FIELD OF MEDICINE DURING RENAISSANCE PERIOD

## Leonardo-da-Vinci

His research centered around his desire to learn more about how the human brain processes visual and sensory information and how that connects to the soul.

He was first to demonstrate the ventricles of brain by wax injection and to depict correctly the foetus and its membrane within the uterus. Originally he studied the bones and muscles in relation to art. He pursued his investigation to study the deeper parts of the body, viscera, brain blood vessels and more specially the heart.

He believed that visual information entered the body through the eye and then continued by sending nerve impulses through the optic nerve, and eventually reaching the soul.

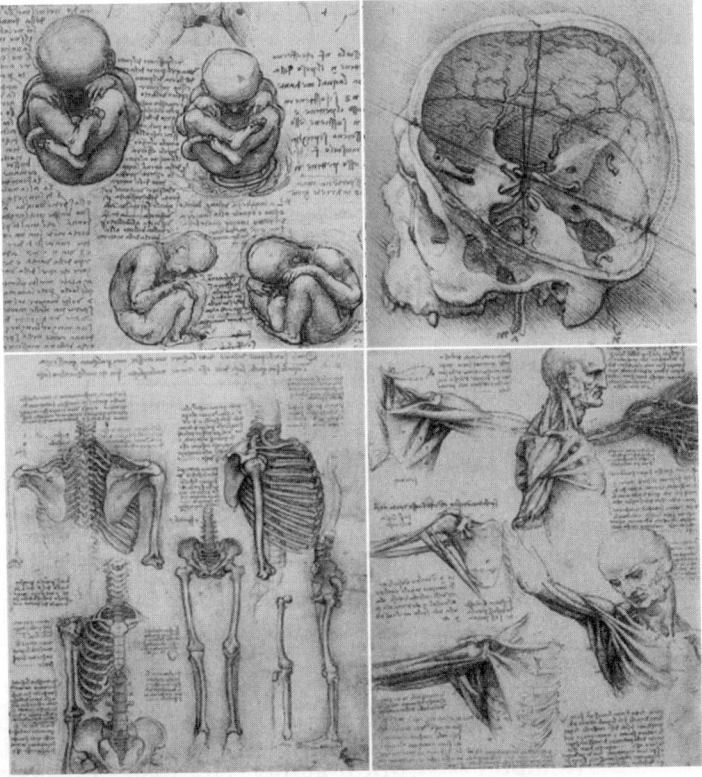

3-D anatomical drawings by Leonardo-da-Vinci

Da-Vinci believed the ancient notion that the soul was housed in the brain.

Leonardo-da-Vinci made his anatomical sketches based on observing and dissecting 30 cadavers. His sketches were very detailed and included organs, muscles of superior extremity, the hand, and the skull. Leonardo was well known for his three-dimensional drawings. His anatomical drawings were not found until 380 years after his death! Though his artwork was widely observed before, some of his original research was not made public until the 20th century.

### Paracelsus

He was the most disputed person of the time in the 16th century. His father was a physician and he practiced in a number of mining towns. Paracelsus had chemical view of life. In his work he has mentioned 'paramirum sulphur, mercury, salt'—meaning sulphur burns, mercury becomes smoke and salt becomes ash. According to his principle all diseases depend upon the maladjustment of the three.

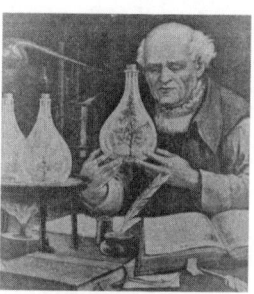

Paracelsus

### Ambroise Paré

He was a French surgeon, anatomist and an inventor of surgical instruments. He was a military surgeon during the French campaigns in Italy in period 1533–36. He reformed surgical practice when he started using ligatures to stop bleeding, rather than painful procedure of cauterization. For the ligatures of arteries, he used silk threads to tie up the arteries of amputated limbs to try to stop the bleeding. As antiseptics had not yet been invented this method led to an increased fatality rate and was abandoned by medical professionals of that time. Additionally, Paré set up a school for midwives in Paris and designed artificial limbs.

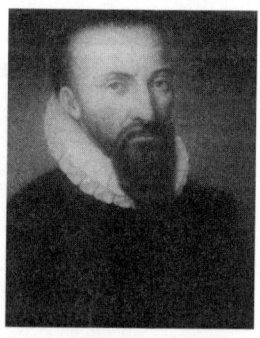

Ambroise Paré

### Andreas Vesalius

He had a background of medical family. He was a professor of anatomy at Padua, Italy in 1537. He had secretly collected a skeleton of a criminal from a gallows (crossbar for hanging criminals) outside the city wall! His dissections of the human body helped to rectify the misconceptions made in ancient times, particularly by Galen, who (for religious reasons) had been able only to study animals such as dogs and monkeys. He wrote many books on anatomy from his observations; his best-known work was 'De Humani Corporis Fabrica', published in 1543, which contained detailed drawings of the human body posed as if alive. Through his figures he represented body in action.

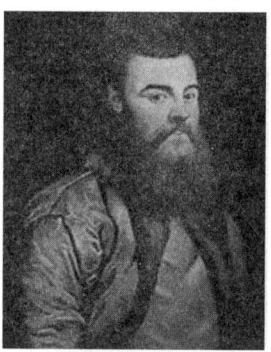

Andreas Vesalius

Vesalius changed how human anatomy was viewed and researched. He is considered a legacy in the medical world.

### William Harvey

He was an English medical doctor-physicist, known for his contributions in heart and blood movement. In 1626, he made a huge breakthrough by studying dying dogs, showing that the heart pumped blood around the body and that the heart had two distinct beating halves. This discovery that blood circulated around the body changed medical practice and finally sounded the death knell for the harmful practice of bloodletting by barber-surgeons. It also

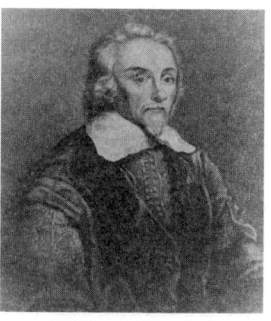

William Harvey

showed that the body contained specialized systems with different functions, all of which worked together in coordination to maintain life, a discovery that led to belief that the body was little more than a machine.

### Hieronymus Fabricius

He was an anatomist and surgeon who prepared a human and animal anatomy atlas 'Tabulae Pictae'. This work includes illustrations from many different artists and Fabricius is credited for providing a turning point in anatomical illustration.

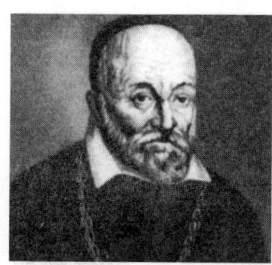

Hieronymus Fabricius

### Pierre Franco

He was first person to perform a subpubic lithotomy. He wrote an article on hernia. He achieved great success in operating cataract.

### Gabriel Fallopius

He is credited for his discovery of *aqueduct* and *fallopian tubes* during the period 1526–62.

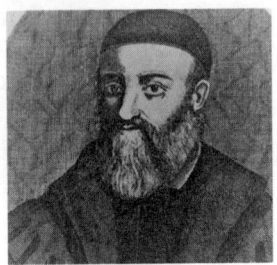

Gabriel Fallopius

### Bartolomeus Eustachius

He was Head of the Department of Anatomy at Rome. He was the first one to accurately illustrate *thoracic duct, cillary muscles*, details of *fascial muscles, larnyx and kidney.*

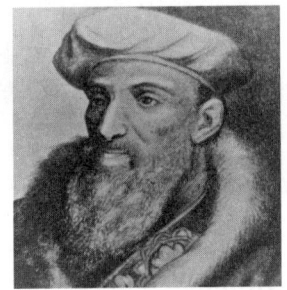

Bartolomeus Eustachius

## MODERN MEDICINE (18th Century Onwards)

18th century was harbinger of the Age of Enlightenment. The practice of medicine changed in the face of rapid advances in science, as well as new approaches by physicians. In hospitals, doctors began much more systematic analysis of patients' symptoms for diagnosis. Among the more powerful new techniques were anaesthesia, and the development of both antiseptic and aseptic operating theatres. Effective cures were developed for certain endemic infectious diseases. However, the decline in many of the lethal diseases was due more to improvements in public health and nutrition than advances in medicine.

Medicine was revolutionized in the 19th century and beyond by advances in chemistry, laboratory techniques, and equipment. Old ideas of infectious disease epidemiology were gradually replaced by advances in bacteriology and virology.

In 1798, **Edward Jenner's** work on vaccinations, in particular for smallpox was a landmark in the development of preventative medicine.

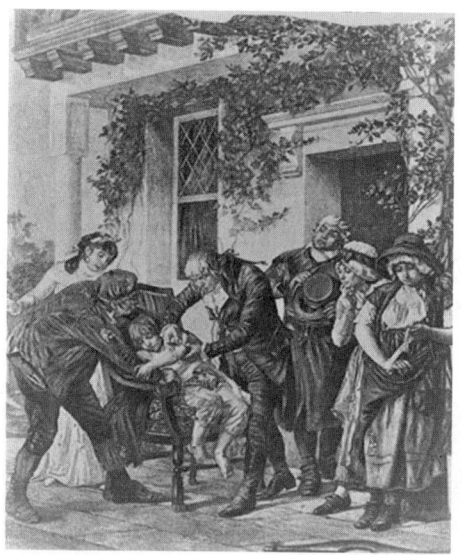

Edward Jenner testing smallpox vaccine

In 1864, **Louis Pasteur** proved that germs caused disease. He proved there are germs in the air by sterilizing water and keeping it in a flask that didn't allow airborne particles to enter. This stayed sterile—but sterilized water kept in an open flask bred microbes again.

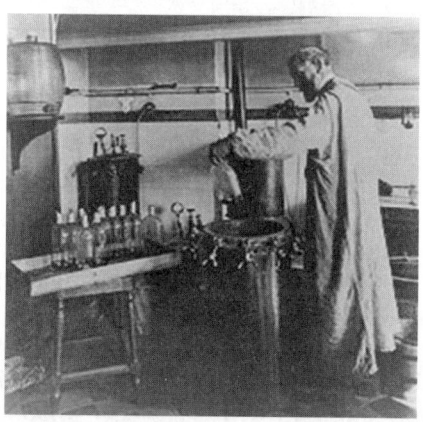

Louis Pasteur working in his laboratory on 'germs'

In 1884 , **Robert Koch** discovered that bacteria caused diseases.

In 1880, **Charles Chamberland** discovered that injecting weakened germs inoculated the patient against that disease.

By 1900, scientists had discovered that viruses also caused diseases and malaria was carried by mosquitoes.

Researchers developed inoculations against rabies (1885), tuberculosis (1906) and diphtheria (1913).

In 1909, the German scientist **Paul Ehrlich** discovered that the chemical Salvarsan 606 cured syphilis.

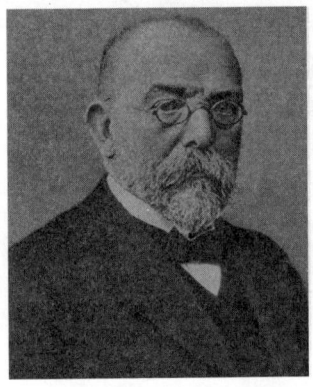
Robert Koch

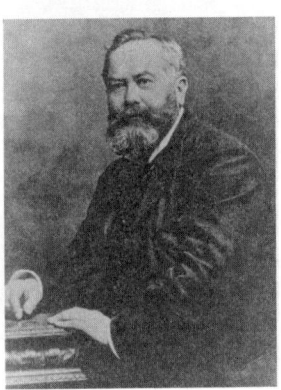
Charles Chamberland

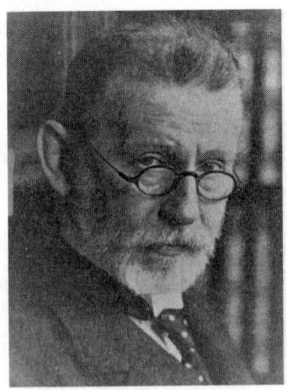
Paul Ehrlich

At this point of history, it was for the first time that a patient had the prospect of going into hospital, undergoing an operation without pain or infection, and surviving!

The development of anaesthetics such as chloroform, discovered by **James Simpson** in 1847, greatly improved the success rate of surgery. Though initially anaesthetics weren't popular as they were uncomfortable for patients. Moreover, some doctors believed that pain was good for healing. Also at that time people didn't understand how they worked and the side effects on the body were not properly recognised. The final breakthrough came when Queen Victoria accepted the use of chloroform as an anaesthetic during the delivery of her eighth child.

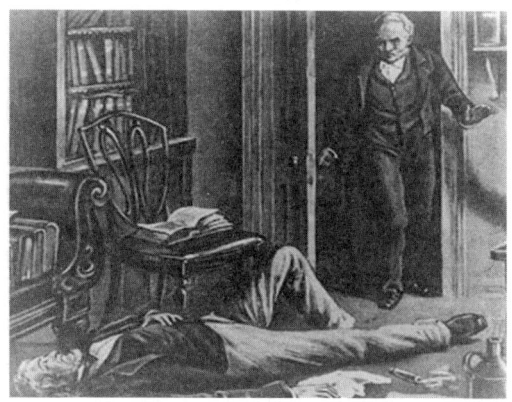

James Simpson experimenting with chloroform for anaesthesia

Until Louis Pasteur's pioneering work on germ theory in the 1860s, surgeons left wounds unprotected. They reused bandages and rarely washed their hands or surgical equipment before operations. In 1864, **Joseph Lister** (Listerine mouth-wash named after him) introduced an antiseptic spray that by 1866, reduced the death rate in patients by 45.7%. Antiseptic methods led to aseptic surgery and the introduction of sterile instruments in operating theatres. By 1898 rubber gloves were used and surgeon's hands were scrubbed clean beforehand.

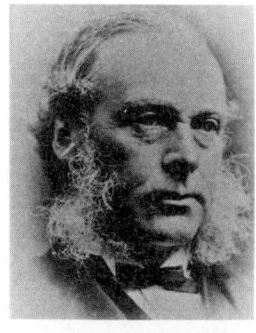

After 1860, as a result of the work of **Florence Nightingale,** there was upliftment in standards of nursing in Britain and also improvements in cleanliness in hospitals. She also worked for establishment of nursing training schools. By 1900, there were 64,000 trained nurses.

Joseph Lister— Listerine mouthwash named after him

By the end of nineteenth century, surgeons were regularly doing successful internal operations, e.g. appendectomies. **X-rays** (which were discovered in 1895) allowed doctors to see inside the body helping in the diagnosis and treatment of patients. Later **ultrasonic imaging, CT scanning, MR scanning** and other imaging methods became available.

In 1854, **John Snow** discovered the connection between contaminated water and cholera by plotting the course of a cholera outbreak in the Broad Street area of London. He noticed that all the victims used the same water pump. When he removed the handle from the pump, the epidemic ended.

There is no time when it is 'good' to become ill, but the 20th century was a much better time to be ill than any previous period in history. By 1991, the average life expectancy of a man in Britain was 73, and that of a woman, 78!

Based on following spectacular scientific discoveries, doctors now understand the human body like never before.

- **Willem Einthoven** in Holland invented the electrocardiograph, or heart monitor in the early 1900s.
- **Karl Landsteiner** in Austria discovered blood groups in 1901.
- The discovery of **penicillin by Alexander Fleming.** Inspired by his work, **Florey and Chain** in the 1930s learned how to mass-produce the penicillin—the first antibiotic.
- The electron microscope was developed in 1931.
- **Francis Crick and James Watson** in Britain discovered the molecular structure of DNA in 1953.
- **Leroy Stevens** in America discovered **stem cells** in 1953.
- **Godfrey Hounsfield** in Britain invented the CAT scanner (a powerful X-ray machine that provides a cross-section of the human body) in 1972.
- **The Human Genome project** mapped all the 40,000 genes in the human body in the 1990s.
- The discovery of vitamins allowed doctors to cure diseases such as rickets.
- In 1922, the first clinical trials of injected insulin saved people with diabetes.
- British surgeon, **Archibald McIndoe,** did the **first plastic surgery** on the faces of disfigured airmen in the 1940s. They were nicknamed the 'Guinea Pig Club'.

- South African surgeon, **Christian Barnard**, performed the first heart transplant in 1967.
- **Louise Brown** became the first **'test-tube baby'** in 1978.
- **Laparoscopic surgery** or **'keyhole surgery'** technique, which avoided using large surgical cuts, became popular in the 1990s.
- **Remote surgery** is another recent development, with the Lindbergh operation in 2001 as a ground-breaking example.
- **Oral rehydration therapy** has been extensively used since 1970s to treat cholera and other diarrhea-inducing infections.
- The sexual revolution included taboo-breaking research in human sexuality such as the invention of hormonal contraception and the normalization of abortion and homosexuality in many countries. Family planning has promoted a demographic transition in most of the world. With threatening sexually transmitted infections use of barrier contraception has become imperative.
- Genetics have advanced with the discovery of the DNA molecule, **genetic mapping** and **gene therapy**. Stem cell research took off in the 2000s, **with stem cell therapy** as a promising method.
- **Evidence-based medicine** is a modern concept, not introduced to literature until the 1990s.
- **Prosthetics** have improved.

  In 1958, Arne Larsson in Sweden became the first patient to depend on an artificial cardiac pacemaker. He died in 2001 at age 86. Lightweight materials as well as neural prosthetics emerged in the end of the 20th century.
- Open-heart surgery was introduced for the first time in 1925. Cardiac surgery was further revolutionized 1948 onwards.
- In **1954, Joseph Murray**, **J. Hartwell Harrison** and others accomplished the first kidney transplantation. Transplantations of other organs, such as heart, liver and pancreas, were also introduced during the late 20th century. The first partial face transplant was performed in 2005, and the first full one in 2010.
- By the end of the 20th century, microtechnology had been used to create tiny robotic devices to assist microsurgery using micro-video and fiberoptic cameras to view internal tissues during surgery with minimally invasive practices.

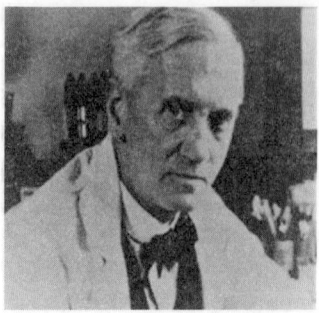
Alexander Fleming

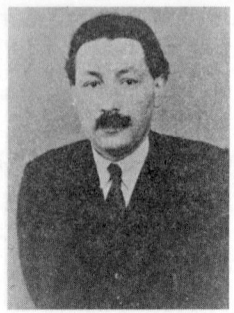
Ernst Chain

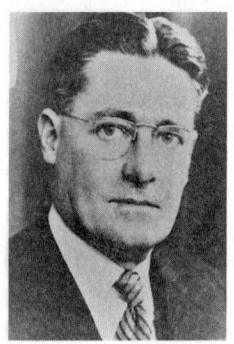
Howard Florey

All three were awarded Nobel Prize for discovery and manufacture of Penicillin in 1945.

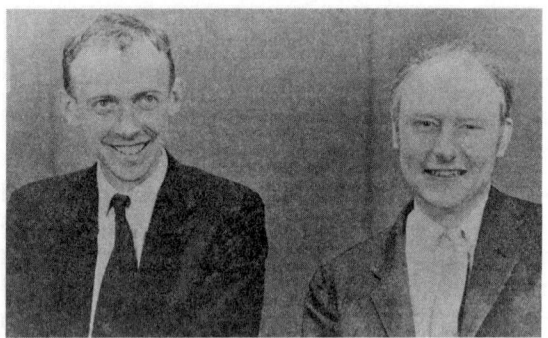
Watson and Crick

Watson, Crick, and **Maurice Wilkins** received '1962 Nobel Prize in Physiology or medicine' for their discoveries concerning the molecular structure of **nucleic acids**.

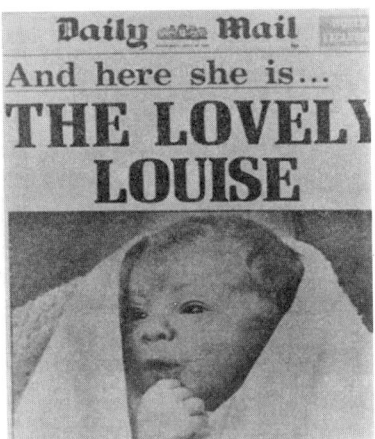

First Test Tube Baby—Louise Brown arrived in 1978

## WOMEN AS PHYSICIANS AFTER THE ADVENT OF ERA OF MODERN MEDICINE

It was very difficult for women to become doctors in any field in early nineteenth century. It was a pity that women doctors, if any, were paid less than their male counterparts and sometimes even less than male factory workers!

### Elizabeth Blackwell and Elizabeth Garrett Anderson

These two british women, born in 1821 and 1836 respectively, were instrumental not only in the emancipation of women but also for admitting of women to the medical profession.

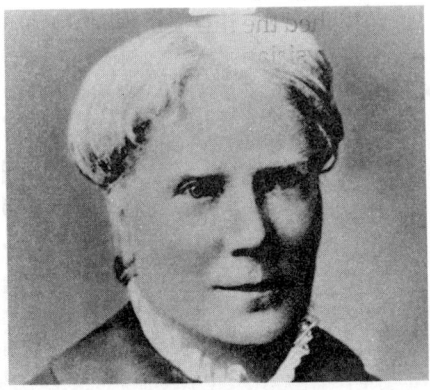

Elizabeth Blackwell

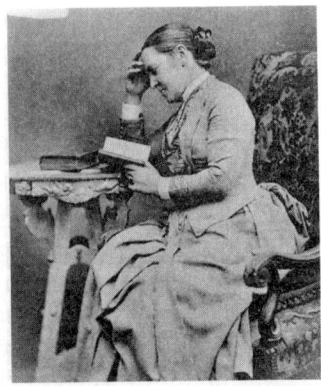

Elizabeth Garrett Anderson

While Blackwell viewed medicine as a means for social and moral reform, her student **Mary Putnam Jacobi** (1842–1906) focused on curing disease.

Even after Blackwell had broken the barrier to medical education, women students faced obstacles like that of exclusion from hospital training and practice.

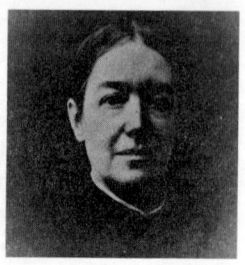

Mary Putnam Jacobi

## UNFORGETTABLE INDIAN NAMES IN THE FIELD OF MEDICINE

### From History

**Bidhan Chandra Roy** (1 July 1882 – 1 July 1962) was an eminent Indian physician, educationist, philanthropist, freedom fighter and politician who served as the Chief Minister of West Bengal from 1948 until his death in 1962. He is often considered the Maker of Modern West Bengal due to his key role in the founding of several institutions and five eminent cities, Durgapur, Kalyani, Bidhannagar, Ashokenagar and Habra. He is one of the few people in history to have obtained FRCS and MRCP degrees simultaneously.

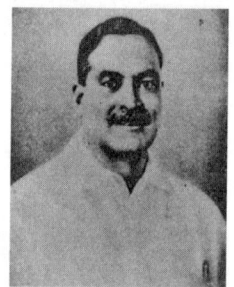

Bidhan Chandra Roy

After completing his matriculation from Patna Collegiate School in 1897, he obtained his IA degree from Presidency College, Calcutta and BA from Patna College with Honors in Mathematics. After completing his graduation in mathematics, he applied for admission to the IIEST formerly BESU and the Calcutta Medical College. He completed his postgraduation in just 2 years and 3 months, and in May 1911 accomplished the rare feat of becoming a member of the Royal College of Physicians and a fellow of the Royal College of Surgeons simultaneously. He returned home from England in 1911.

Immediately after graduation, Roy joined the Provincial Health Service. He exhibited immense dedication and hard work, and would even serve as a nurse when necessary. In his free time he practiced privately, charging a nominal fee.

Following his return from England after postgraduation, he taught at the Calcutta Medical College, and later at the Campbell Medical School and the Carmichael Medical College.

Dr Roy believed that 'Swaraj' (the call to action for India's freedom) would remain a dream unless the people were healthy and strong in mind and body. He made contributions to the organisation of medical education. He played an important role in the establishment of the Jadavpur TB Hospital, Chittaranjan Seva Sadan, Kamala Nehru Memorial Hospital, Victoria Institution (College), and Chittaranjan Cancer Hospital. The Chittaranjan Seva Sadan for women and children was opened in 1926. Women were unwilling to come to the hospital initially, but due to Dr Roy and his team's hard work, the Seva Sadan was embraced by women of all classes and communities. He opened a center for training women in nursing and social work.

In 1942, Rangoon fell to Japanese bombing and caused an exodus from Calcutta fearing Japanese insurgency. Dr Roy was serving as the Vice-Chancellor of the University of Calcutta. He acquired air-raid shelters for schools and college students to have their classes in, and provided relief for students, teachers and employees alike. In recognition for his efforts, the Doctorate of Science was conferred upon him in 1944.

He believed that the youth of India would determine the future of the nation. He felt that the youth must not take part in strikes and fasts but should study and commit themselves to social work.

The nation honoured him with the Bharat Ratna on 4 February 1961. On 1 July 1962, his 80th birthday, after treating his morning patients and discharging affairs of the State, he took a copy of the 'Brahmo Geet' and sang a piece from it. Few hours later he died at midday past three.

In India, the National Doctors' Day is celebrated in his memory every year on 1 July. The BC Roy National Award was instituted in 1962 in Dr. Roy's memory and has been awarded annually since 1976. The award recognizes excellent contributions in the areas of medicine, politics, science, philosophy, literature and arts. The Dr BC Roy Memorial Library and Reading Room for Children in the Children's Book Trust, New Delhi, was opened in 1967.

**Rai Bahadur Sir Upendranath Brahmachari (19 December 1873–6 February 1946)** was an Indian scientist and a leading medical practitioner of his time. He synthesized Urea Stibamine (carbostibamide) in 1922 and determined that it was an effective substitute for the other antimony-containing compounds in the treatment of Kala-azar (Visceral leishmaniasis) which is caused by a protozoon, *Leishmania donovani*. His discovery led to the saving of thousands of lives in India, particularly in the erstwhile province of

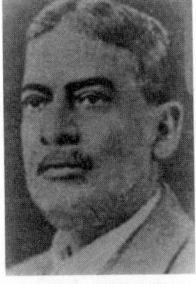

Upendranath
Brahmachari

Assam, where several villages were completely depopulated by the devastating disease. The achievement of Brahmachari was a milestone in successful application of science in medical treatment in the years before arrival of antibiotics, when there were few specific drugs, including quinine for malaria, iron for anaemia, digitalis for heart diseases and arsenic compounds for syphilis. Most other ailments were treated symptomatically by palliative methods. Urea Stibamine was thus a significant addition to the arsenal of specific medicines.

Upendranath Brahmachari was born on 19 December 1873 in Sardanga village near Purbasthali, District Burdwan of West Bengal, India. His father, Nilmony Brahmachari, was a physician in East Indian Railways. His mother's name was Saurabh Sundari Devi. He completed his early education from Eastern Railways Boys' High School, Jamalpur. In 1893, he passed BA degree from Hooghly Mohsin College with honours in Mathematics and Chemistry. Thereafter he went to study Medicine with Higher Chemistry. He passed his master's degree in 1894 from the Presidency College, Kolkata. In MB Examination of 1900 of the University of Calcutta, he stood first in Medicine and in Surgery for which he received Goodeve and Macleod awards. He obtained his MD degree in 1902, and was awarded a PhD degree in 1904, for his research paper on "Studies in Haemolysis" both from the University of Calcutta.

Brahmachari joined the Provincial Medical Service in September 1899 and appointed as a teacher of pathology and Materia Medica, and physician in the Dacca Medical School in 1901. In 1905, he was appointed as a teacher in Medicine and Physician at the Campbell Medical School (now Nilratan Sircar Medical College and Hospital), Calcutta, where he carried out most of his work on Kala-azar and made his monumental discovery of Urea Stibamine. In 1923, he joined as Additional Physician in the Medical College Hospital. He retired from the government service as a physician in 1927. After retirement from the government service Brahmachari joined the Carmichael Medical College in Kolkata as Professor of Tropical Diseases. He also served the National Medical Institute, in-charge of its Tropical Disease Ward. He was also the Head of the Department of Biochemistry and Honorary Professor of Biochemistry at the University College of Science, Calcutta.

Brahmachari played an important part in the formation of the world's second Blood Bank in Kolkata in 1939. He was the

Chairman of the Blood Transfusion Service of Bengal. He was the Vice-President of the St. John Ambulance Association of the Bengal branch and also its President. He was the first Indian to become the Chairman of the Managing Body of the Indian Red Cross Society of the Bengal Branch. For his achievements, he received many awards, including the Griffith Memorial Prize of the University of Calcutta, the Minto Medal by the Calcutta School of Tropical Medicine and Hygiene (1921) and the Sir William Jones Medal by the Asiatic Society of Bengal. He was awarded the title of Rai Bahadur and awarded the Kaisar-i-Hind Gold Medal, 1st Class by the Governor General Lord Lytton (1924). In 1934, he was conferred a Knighthood by the British Government (1934). Brahmachari was a nominee for the Nobel Prize in 1929 in the category of physiology and medicine. The Kolkata Municipal Corporation renamed Loudon Street the Dr UN Brahmachari Street.

**Dr Dwarkanath Kotnis** was born in a lower middle class family on October 10, 1910 in Sholapur, Mumbai. A vivacious kid by nature, Dr Kotnis forever aspired to become a doctor. After completing his graduation in medicine from GS Medical College, Bombay, he went on to pursue his post-graduation internship. However, he shelved his postgraduation plans when he got the chance to join the medical aid mission to China. In 1937, the communist General Zhu De requested Jawaharlal Nehru

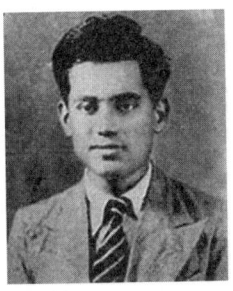

Dwarkanath Kotnis

to send Indian physicians to China during the Second Sino-Japanese War to help the soldiers. A medical team of five doctors, including Dr Kotnis was sent as the part of Indian Medical Mission Team in September 1938. After the war, all other doctors except Dr Kotnis, returned back to India. Dr Kotnis decided to stay back and serve at the military base. Dr Kotnis made China his home and joined the Communist Party of China in July 1942. He also worked as a lecturer for sometime in the Military area at the Dr Bethune Hygiene School. He took over the post of the first president of the Bethune International Peace Hospital after Dr Norman Bethune passed away. Due to inclement weather in China, inadequate diet, and enormous work strain, Dr Kotnis passed away following a sudden seizure attack in December 1942 at an early age of 32.

Dr Kotnis' major contribution was his selfless service to the Chinese soldiers in the battlefield during the Second Sino-Japanese War. He had the heart to stay back in China, even when his colleagues left, just for serving the wounded soldiers during the war. He was fondly dubbed as 'Black Mother' by the Chinese villagers. Because of his loyalty, the young Indian doctor became a legendary figure in China and was honored by China with a gold medal during Sino-Japan war of 1938, for saving thousands of Chinese lives. His role in solidifying relations between China and India has been humungous.

## WOMEN APPLAUDABE AS DOCTORS

**Anandibai Gopalrao Joshi** (31 March 1865–26 February 1887) was the first woman from the erstwhile Bombay presidency of India to study and graduate with a 2-year degree in Western Medicine in the United States.

Originally named Yamuna, Joshi was born and raised in Kalyan, Maharashtra, where her family had previously been landlords before experiencing financial losses. As per the practice at that time she was married at the age of nine to Gopalrao Joshi, a widower almost twenty years older than her. After marriage, Yamuna's husband renamed her 'Anandi'. Gopalrao Joshi worked as a postal clerk in Kalyan and later transferred to Kolkata (Calcutta). He was the man to encourage her study medicine. He was so obsessed with his wife's education that he would abuse and beat her. So much so that one day when he found her cooking in kitchen he went into fits of rage. At the age of fourteen, Anandibai gave birth to a boy, but the child lived only for ten days for lack of medical care. This proved to be a turning point in Anandi's life and inspired her to become a physician.

In 1880, Gopalrao sent a letter to Royal Wilder, a well-known American missionary, stating his wife's interest in studying medicine in the United States and inquiring about a suitable post in the US for himself. Wilder published the correspondence in his Princeton's Missionary Review. Theodicia Carpenter, a resident of Roselle, New Jersey, happened to read it while waiting to see her dentist. Impressed by both Anandibai's desire to study medicine, and Gopalrao's support for his wife, she wrote to Anandibai. Carpenter and Anandibai developed a close friendship and came to refer to each other as 'aunt' and 'niece.' Later, Carpenter hosted Anandibai in Rochelle during her stay in the US.

On learning of Joshis' plans to pursue higher education in the West, orthodox Indian society opposed them very strongly. Anandibai addressed the community at Serampore College Hall, in West Bengal , explaining her decision to go to America and obtain a medical degree. She discussed the hostility and ill-treatment she and her husband were facing. She stressed the need for female doctors in India, emphasizing that Hindu women could better serve as physicians to Hindu women. Her speech received publicity, and financial contributions started pouring in from all over India.

Anandibai travelled to New York from Kolkata (Calcutta) by ship. In New York, Theodicia Carpenter received her in June 1883. Anandibai got herself enrolled in Woman's Medical College of Pennsylvania.

Anandibai began her medical training at age 19. While she was in India she had suffered from weakness, constant headaches, occasional fever, and sometimes breathlessness. In America, her health worsened because of the cold weather and unfamiliar diet. She contracted tuberculosis. Nevertheless, she graduated with an MD in March of 1886. The topic of her thesis was 'Obstetrics among the Aryan Hindoos.' On her graduation, Queen Victoria sent her a congratulatory message.

In late 1886, Anandibai returned to India, receiving a grand welcome. The princely state of Kolhapur appointed her as the

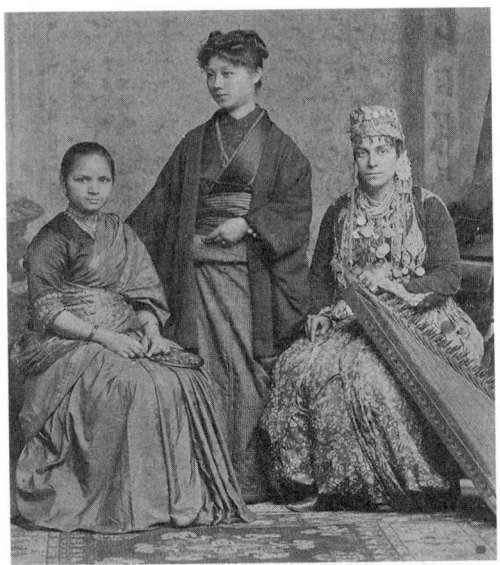

Woman's Medical College of Pennsylvania in 1886

Anandibai Joshi, from India (left) with Kei Okami, Japan (center) and Sabat Islambooly, from Syria (right). All three completed their medical studies and each of them was the first woman from their respective countries to obtain a degree in Western Medicine.

physician-in-charge of the female ward of the local Albert Edward Hospital.

Anandibai died of tuberculosis early the next year on 26 February 1887 before turning 22. Her death was mourned throughout India. Her ashes were sent to Theodicia Carpenter, who placed them in her family cemetery with inscription stating that Anandi Joshi was a Hindu Brahmin girl, the first Indian woman to receive education abroad and to obtain a medical degree.

**Kadambani** was born in a liberal family during the British Raj on 18 July 1861 at Bhagalpur, Bihar.

She studied medicine at the Calcutta Medical College and was awarded graduate degree in 1886. At that she became one of the two Indian women doctors who qualified to practice Western Medicine, Anandi Gopal Joshi being the other. (One more Indian woman by the name of Abala Bose passed entrance in 1881 but was refused admission to the medical college and went to Madras to study medicine but never graduated!)

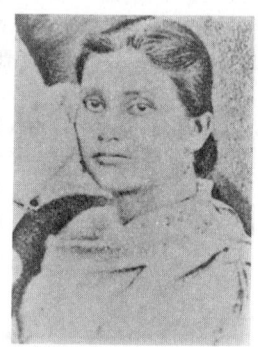

Kadambani Ganguly

Battling stereotypes and refusing to fall into the norm of marriage and family-rearing Ganguly travelled overseas to the UK and returned home only after she had LRCP, LRCS, and GFPS degrees attached to her name. Garnering a better reputation among her male counterparts and superiors, she was offered a job with Lady Dufferin Hospital, Kolkata, following which she began her own practice. Her work was the stepping stone for women aspiring for a career in medicine and was responsible for the countless numbers she inspired to join in the same.

## ONGOING JOURNEY

The preceding writing sundoubtedly prove that history of medicine is endlessly fascinating. It gives an insight as to how early civilizations coped with health problems. This information contributes to our present understanding of medicine and healing.

Every human civilization developed a system of medicine, based on material medica, spells, incantations, magic and rituals. Each has progressed from primitive stage to a regular system of medicine. To maintain good health, cure diseases, and to care for wounds and broken bones was as important to our ancestors as it is to us today and every civilization made best endeavors to keep its population healthy. Over the times, as the human civilizations advanced, the disease pattern changed and so changed the pattern of practice of medicine.

*"We shall free medicine from its worst errors. Not by following that which those of old taught, but by our own observation of nature, confirmed by extensive practice and long experience."* —Paracelsus, 1530

Very aptly said by Paracelsus. Learning from history, today doctors stress on healthy living, prevention of disease, personal and social hygiene and not merely the cure of diseases. Moreover, as a result of globalization, today we are exposed to various patterns of medicine and are in beneficial situation of availing best from each pattern of medicine.

I had started this enthralling saga of man's struggle against disease from prehistoric times and waded out of the history to doctors presently creating history from our own country. Now at this point I wish to pause. I leave it entirely to my readers to dive into ocean of history to depths in accordance to their individual level of inquisitiveness. Following is a list of relevant books which can be referred to for further reading.

# Appendix 2

# Hippocratic Oath

*Nitin Ashok John*

## HIPPOCRATIC OATH: CLASSICAL VERSION

I swear by Apollo Physician and Asclepius and Hygieia and Panaceia and all the Gods and Goddesses, making them my witnesses, that I will fulfill according to my ability and judgment this oath and this covenant:

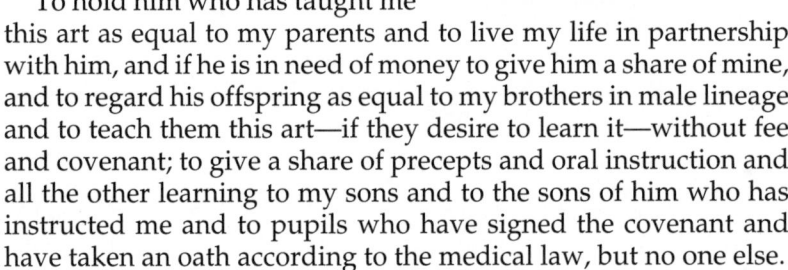

To hold him who has taught me this art as equal to my parents and to live my life in partnership with him, and if he is in need of money to give him a share of mine, and to regard his offspring as equal to my brothers in male lineage and to teach them this art—if they desire to learn it—without fee and covenant; to give a share of precepts and oral instruction and all the other learning to my sons and to the sons of him who has instructed me and to pupils who have signed the covenant and have taken an oath according to the medical law, but no one else.

I will apply dietetic measures for the benefit of the sick according to my ability and judgment; I will keep them from harm and injustice.

I will neither give a deadly drug to anybody who asked for it, nor will I make a suggestion to this effect. Similarly I will not give to a woman an abortive remedy. In purity and holiness I will guard my life and my art.

I will not use the knife, not even on sufferers from stone, but will withdraw in favor of such men as are engaged in this work.

Whatever houses I may visit, I will come for the benefit of the sick, remaining free of all intentional injustice, of all mischief and in particular of sexual relations with both female and male persons, be they free or slaves.

What I may see or hear in the course of the treatment or even outside of the treatment in regard to the life of men, which on no account one must spread abroad, I will keep to myself, holding such things shameful to be spoken about.

If I fulfill this oath and do not violate it, may it be granted to me to enjoy life and art, being honored with fame among all men for all time to come; if I transgress it and swear falsely, may the opposite of all this be my lot.

## HIPPOCRATIC OATH: MODERN VERSION

**Hippocratic oath:** Medical Ethics and Declaration of Geneva.

### Medical Ethics

The general principle mentioned in the Hippocratic Oath has been updated by the World Medical Association. The modernized version of the Hippocratic Oath is the Declaration of Geneva, of September 1948, and the International Code of Medical Ethics, as adopted by the General Assembly of the World Medical Association held in London, in October, 1948.

### THE DECLARATION OF GENEVA

At the time of being admitted as a member of the medical profession.
- I solemnly pledge as a member of the medical profession.
- I will give due respect and gratitude to my teachers.
- I will practice my profession with the consideration.
- The health of my patient will be my first consideration.
- I will respect the secrets which are confided in me.
- I will maintain by all means in my power, the honour and noble traditions of the medical profession.
- My colleagues will be my brothers.
- I will not permit consideration of religion, nationality, race, party, politics or social standing to intervene between my duty and my patients.
- I will maintain the utmost respect for human life since the time of conception.
- Even under threat, I will not use my medical knowledge contrary to the laws of humanity.

I make these promises solemnly, freely and upon my honour.

# Further Reading

## MODULE 1.1: What does it Mean to be a Doctor?

1. Adler HM. The sociophysiology of caring in the doctor—patient relationship. *J Gen Intern Med* 2002; 17: 883–90.
2. Aharony L, Strasser S. "Patient satisfaction: What we know about and what we still need to explore." *Medical Care Review* 1993; 50(1): 49–79.
3. Anderson L, Dedrick R. Development of the trust in physician scale: A measure to assess interpersonal trust in patient-physician relationship. *Psychology Rep* 1990; 67: 1091–100.
4. Becker JL, Milad MP, Klock SC. Burnout, depression, and career satisfaction: cross-sectional study of obstetrics and gynecology residents. *Am J Obstet Gynecol* 2006; 195: 1444–9.
5. Benson D. Personal communication. Bethesda, MD: National Library of Medicine; Nov, 2014.
6. Berger D. Corruption ruins the doctor-patient relationship in India. *BMJ* 2014; 348: g3169.
7. Bertman SL, Marks SC. Humanities in medical education: rationale and resources for the dissection laboratory. *Med Educ* 1985; 19: 374–81.
8. Bhardwaj A, Chopra M, Mithra P, Singh A, Siddiqui A, Rajesh DR. Current status of knowledge, attitudes and practices towards healthcare ethics among doctors and nurses from Northern India—A Multicentric Study. *Pravara Med Rev* 2014; 6: 4–8.
9. Bolhuis S. Toward process-oriented teaching for self-directed lifelong learning: a multidimensional perspective. *Learning Instruction* 2003; 13: 327–47.
10. Carlton KH. Redefining continuing education delivery. *Computers Nurs* 1997; 15: 17–18.
11. Cassell EJ. The Healer's Art: A New Approach to the Doctor Patient Relationship. New York: Lippencott; 1976. pp. 47–83.
12. Chatterjee C, Srinivasan V. Ethical issues in healthcare sector in India. *IIMB Manag Rev* 2013;25:49–62.
13. Cote L, Leclerc H. How clinical teachers perceive the doctor-patient relationship and themselves as role models. *Acad Med* 2000; 75: 1117–24.
14. Dash SK. Medical ethics, duties and medical negligence awareness among the practitioners in a teaching medical college, hospital—A survey. *J Indian Acad Forensic Med* 2010; 32: 153–6.

15. David RA, Rhee M. "The impact of language as a barrier to effective healthcare in an under served urban hispanic community." *The Mount Sinai Journal of Medicine* 1998; 65 (5–6): 393–7.

16. Davis DA, Thomson MA, Oxman AD, Haynes RB. Changing physician performance. A systematic review of the effect of continuing medical education strategies. *JAMA* 1995; 274: 700–5.

17. de Groot J, van Hoek M, Hoedemaekers C, Hoitsma A, Smeets W, Vernooij-Dassen M, et al. Decision making on organ donation: The dilemmas of relatives of potential brain dead donors. *BMC Med Ethics* 2015; 16: 64.

18. Editorial. The Indian Medical Council (Professional conduct, Etiquitte and Ethics) Regulations 2002. *Indian Journal of Medical Ethics* Nov 2016; (S1) V. 10, N. 3 P. 66.

19. Emanuel EJ, Dubler NN. Preserving the physician—patient relationship in the era of managed care. *JAMA* 1995; 273: 323–9.

20. Epstein RM, Hundert EM. Defining and assessing professional competence. *JAMA* 2002; 287: 226–35.

21. Gallagher TH, Levinson W. A prescription for protecting the doctor—patient relationship. *Am J Manage Care* 2004; 10: 61–8.

22. Good BJ. Medicine, Rationalitiy, and Experience: An Anthropological Perspective. Cambridge: Cambridge University Press, 1994.

23. Gordon C, Bcresin EV. The doctor-patient relationship. In: Stern TA, Fava M, Wilens TE, et al., editors. Massachusetts General Hospital Comprehensive Clinical Psychiatry. 2nd ed. Philadelphia, PA: Elsevier Health Sciences; 2016. pp. 1–7.

24. Hafferty FW. Cadaver stories and the emotional socialization of medical students. *J Health Soc Behav* 1988; 29: 344–56.

25. Hafferty FW. Into the Valley: Death and the Socialization of Medical Students. New Haven: Yale University Press, 1991.

26. Hariharan S, Jonnalagadda R, Walrond E, Moseley H. Knowledge, attitudes and practice of healthcare ethics and law among doctors and nurses in *Barbados. BMC Med Ethics* 2006; 7: E7.

27. Heard SR, Schiller G, Aitken M, Fergie C, McCready Hall L. Continuous quality improvement: educating towards a culture of clinical governance. *Qual Healthcare* 2001; 10 (suppl 2): S70–S78.

28. Hojat M, Gonnella JS, Erdmann JB, Veloski JJ, Xu G. Primary care and non-primary care physicians: a longitudinal study of their similarities. *Acad Med* 1995; 70: S17–28.

29. Howie JG, Heaney DJ, Maxwell M, Walker JJ. Quality at general practice consultations; cross-sectional survey. *Br Med J* 1999; 319: 738–43.

30. Inui TS, Carter WB, Kukull WA, et al. Outcome-based doctor-patient interaction analysis: I. comparison of techniques. *Med Care* 1982; 20(6): 535–49.

31. Lella JW, Pawluch D. Medical students and the cadaver in social and cultural context. In: Lock M, Gordon DR, eds. Biomedicine Examined. Dordrecht: Kluwer, 1988: 125–53.

32. Lrvine D. The performance of doctors. I: Professionalism and self regulation in a changing world. *BMJ* 1997 May 24; 314(7093): 1540–2.

33. Mahajan R, Aruldhas BW, Sharma M, Badyal DK, Singh T. Professionalism and ethics: A proposed curriculum for undergraduates. *Int J Appl Basic Med Res* 2016; 6: 157–63.

34. Malvinder S Parmar. ABC of being a good doctor. *BMJ* 2002 Sep 28; 325 (7366): 711.

35. Mandal J, Ponnambath DK, Parija SC. Bioethics: A brief review. *Trop Parasitol* 2017; 7: 5–7.

36. Mazmanian PE, Davis DA. Continuing medical education and the physician as a learner: guide to the evidence. *JAMA* 2002; 288: 1057–60.

37. McCarthy M. Computer and internet: tools for lifelong learning. *J Renal Nutr* 2000; 10: 44–48.

38. Miflin BM, Campbell CB, Price DA. A lesson from the introduction of a problem-based, graduate entry course: the effects of different views of self-direction. *Med Educ* 1999; 33: 801–7.

39. Mueller PS. Incorporating professionalism into medical education: The mayo clinic experience. *Keio J Med* 2009; 58: 133–4.

40. Rameshkumar K. Ethics in medical curriculum; ethics by the teachers for students and society. *Indian J Urol* 2009; 25: 337–9.

41. Ridd M, Shaw A, Lewis G, et al. The patient-doctor relationship: a synthesis of the qualitative literature on patients' perspectives. *Br J Gen Pract* 2009; 59(561): e116- e133.

42. Rosenfield PJ, Jones L. Striking a balance: training medical students to provide empathetic care. *Med Educ* 2004; 38: 927–33.

43. Ruhl DS, Siegal G. Medical malpractice implications of clinical practice guidelines. *Otolaryngol Head Neck Surg* 2017; 157: 175–7.

44. Schotzinger KA, Kirkley Best E. Closure and the cadaver experience: a memorial service for deeded bodies. *Omega J Death Dying* 1987; 18: 217–27.

45. Sharp PA. Meeting global challenges: discovery and innovation through convergence. *Science* 2014 Dec 19; 346 (621).

46. Snyder L. American College of Physicians Ethics, Professionalism, and Human Rights Committee. American college of physicians ethics manual: Sixth edition. *Ann Intern Med* 2012; 156 (1 Pt 2): 73–104.

47. Stewart MA. Effective physician-patient communication and health outcomes: a review. *CMAJ* 1995; 152(9): 1423–33.

48. Street RL, Krupat E, Bell RA, Kravitz RL, Haidet P. Beliefs about control in the physician—patient relationship. *J Gen Intern Med* 2003; 18: 609–16.

49. Szasz TS, Hollender MH. A contribution to the philosophy of medicine: the basic models of the doctor-patient relationship. *AMA Arch Intern Med* 1956; 97(5): 585–92.

50. Wenger E. Communities of Practice: Learning, Meaning, and Identity. Cambridge: Cambridge University Press, 1998

51. Woloshin S, Bickell NA, Schwartz LM, Gany F, Welch G. "Language Barriers in Medicine in the United States." *JAMA* 1995; 273(9): 724–8.

52. Wright SM, Kern DE, Kolodner K, Howard DM, Brancati FL. Attributes of excellent attending-physician role models. *N Engl J Med* 1998; 339: 1986–93.

53. Yoon JD, Rasinski KA, Curlin FA. Moral controversy, directive counsel, and the doctor's role: findings from a national survey of obstetrician-gynecologists. *Acad Med* 2010; 85: 1475–81.

## MODULE 1.2: What does it Mean to be a Patient?

1. Anfossi M, Numico G. Empathy in the doctor-patient relationship. *J Clinoncol* 2004; 22(11): 2258–9.

2. Beck RS, Daughtridge R, Sloane PD. Physician–patient communication in the primary care office: a systematic review. *J Am Board Fam Pract* 2002; 15: 25–38 8.

3. Bellet PS, Maloney MJ. The importance of empathy as an interviewing skill. *JAMA* 1991; 266(13): 1831–2.

4. Bratek A, Bulska W, Bonk M, Seweryn M, Krysta K. Empathy among physicians, medical students and candidates. *Psychiatr Danub* 2015 Sep; 27 Suppl 1: S48–52. 9.

5. Carma L. Bylund Gregory Makoul. Examining Empathy in Medical Encounters: An Observational Study Using the Empathic Communication Coding System. HEALTH COMMUNICATION, 18(2), 123–140.

6. Finset A, Ørnes K. Empathy in the Clinician-Patient Relationship: The Role of Reciprocal Adjustments and Processes of Synchrony. *J Patient Exp* 2017 Jun; 4(2): 64–68. doi: 10.1177/2374373517699271. Epub 2017 May 9. 10.

7. Kraft-Todd GT, Reinero DA, Kelley JM, Heberlein AS, Baer L, Riess H. Empathic Non-verbal behaviour increases ratings of both warmth and competence in a medical context. *PLoS ONE* 2017; 12(5): e0177758. https://doi.org/10.1371/journal.pone.0177758

8. Platt FW, Keller VF. Empathic communication: a teachable and learnable skill. *J Gen Intern Med* 1994; 9(4):222–6.

9. Riess H, Kelley JM, Bailey RW, Dunn EJ, Phillips M. Empathy Training for Resident Physicians: A Randomized Controlled Trial of a Neuroscience-Informed Curriculum. *Journal of General Internal Medicine* 2012; 27(10): 1280–6. pmid: 22549298 7.

10. Teding van Berkhout E, Malouff JM. The efficacy of empathy training: A meta-analysis of randomized controlled trials. *Journal of counseling psychology* 2016; 63(1): 32.

## MODULE 1.3: Doctor-Patient Relationship

1. Arora NK, Finney Rutten LJ, Gustafson DH, Moser R, Hawkins RP. Perceived helpfulness and impact of social support provided by family, friends, and healthcare providers to women newly diagnosed with breast cancer. *Psychooncology* 2007; 16(5): 474–486.

2. Emanuel EJ, Dubler NN. Preserving the physician-patient relationship in the era of managed care. *JAMA* 1995; 273(4): 323–9.

3. Grazier KL, Richardson WC, Martin DP, Diehr P. Factors affecting choice of healthcare plans. *Health Serv Res* 1986; 20(6 pt 1): 659–82.

4. Halpern J. Can the development of practice guidelines safeguard patient values. *J Law Med Ethics* 1995; 23(1): 75–81.

5. Holmström I, Röing M. The relation between patient-centeredness and patient empowerment: a discussion on concepts. *Patient Education and Counseling* 2010; 79(2): 167–72.

6. Mendoza MD, Smith SG, Eder MM, Hickner J. The seventh element of quality: the doctor-patient relationship. *Fam Med* 2011; 43(2): 83–9.

7. Morton KR, Worthly JS, Testerman JK, Mahoney ML. Defining features of moral sensitivity and moral motivation: pathways to moral reasoning in medical students. *J Moral Educ* 2006; 35(3): 387–406.

8. Phillips—Salimi CR, Haase JE, Kooken WC. Connectedness in the context of patient-provider relationships: a concept analysis. *J Adv Nurs* 2012; 68(1): 230–45.

9. Sadati AK, Lankarani KB, Enayat H, Kazerooni AR, Ebrahimzadeh S. Clinical Paternalistic Model and Problematic Situation: A Critical Evaluation of Clinical Counseling. *Journal of Health Sciences and Surveillance System* 2014; 2(2): 78–87.

10. Sadati AK, Tabei SZ, Ebrahimzade N, Zohri M, Argasi H, Lankarani KB. The paradigm model of distorted doctor-patient relationship in SouthernIran: a grounded theory study. *J Med Ethics Hist Med* April. 2016; 9:2.

## MODULE 1.4: The Foundations of Communication 1

1. Attitude, Ethics and Communication competencies for the Indian Medical Graduate—Medical Council of India.

2. Changing medical education—Grant J R and Gale R.

3. Concise principles of Medical Education—Manual of the Medical Education Unit of Chettinad Hospital and Research Institute.

4. Faculty development for teaching and evaluating professionalism: from programme design to curriculum change—Yvonne Steinert, Sylvia Cruess, Richard Cruess and Linda Snell.

5. Improving teaching skills: from interactive classroom to applicable knowledge—PredragVujovic.

6. Incorporating Professionalism into Medical Education: The Mayo Clinic Experience—Paul S. Mueller.
7. Making conflict management a strategic advantage—Kenneth W Thomas.
8. Principles of Medical Education—Tejinder Singh, Piyush Gupta and Daljit Singh.
9. Resource material of the Advanced Course in Medical Education conducted in the Christian Medical College Vellore.
10. Resource material of the Revised Basic Course Workshop conducted in the Christian Medical College Vellore.
11. Shaping strategic changes – Pettigrew A, Ferlie E and Mckee L.
12. Student Learning Preferences and Teaching Implications—Robert J. Murphy, MBA Sarah A Gray, DDS, MS; Sorin R Straja, PhD; Meredith C Bogert, DMD.
13. The integration ladder: a tool for curriculum planning and evaluation—Ronald M Harden.
14. Toolkit for Academic Leaders—Ray Wells.
15. Use of the Kalamazoo essential elements communication checklist in an institutional inter personal and communication skills curriculum-Barbara L. Joyce, PhD Timothy Steenbergh, PhD Eric Scher, MD.
16. WFME global standards of quality improvement.

## MODULE 1.5: Cadaver as Our First Teacher

1. Der Bedrosian J. First-year medical students still rely on cadavers to learn anatomy. John Hopkins Magazine. 2016. Available from: https://hub. jhu.edu//magazine/2016/winter/cadaves-anatomy-medical-school/.
2. Ghosh SK. Human cadaveric dissection: a historical account from ancient Greece to the modern era. *Anat Cell Biol* 2015; 48(3): 153–69.
3. Hehmeyer I, Khan A. Islam's forgotten contributions to medical science. *Can Med Assoc J* 2007 May; 176: 1467–8.
4. Kanter SL, A Silent Mentor. Acad Med 2010;85(3):389.
5. Kantor SL. A silent mentor. *Acad Med* 2010 Mar; 85(3)389.
6. McCall M. The Secret Lives of Cadavers. National Geographic. July 2016. Available from: https://news.nationalgeographic.com/2016/07/body-donation-cadavers-anatomy-medical-eductions/.
7. Merriam-Webster I. Merriam-Webster's collegiate dictionary. Springfield: Merriam-Webster; 2003.
8. Paff M. Teaching and learning moment-artist's statement: my cadaver. *Acad Med* 2009 Jul; 84(7): 829.
9. Savage-Smith E. Attitudes toward dissection in medieval Islam. *J Hist Med Allied Sci* 1995 Jan; 50(1): 67–110.

10. Sawant SP, Shaikh S, De Sousa A. Cadaveric Oath in Anatomy-an integral aspect of bioethics training (Brief Report). *Global Bioethics Enquiry* 2016; 4: 64–6.
11. Shaikh ST. Cadaver dissection in anatomy: the ethical aspect. *Anat Physiol* 2015; 1:S5–7.
12. Sheriff Ds, Sheriff O. The human cadaver: the silent teacher of human anatomy. *Indian J Med Ethics* 2010; 7: 266–8.
13. Sheriff DS. Medical ethics and reverence for life. *Eubios J Asian Int Bioeth* 2003; 13: 224–6.
14. Winkelmann A, Guldner FH. Cadavers as teachers: the dissecting room experience in Thailand. *BMJ* 2004; 329(7480): 1455–7.
15. Wojciech P. Hammer RR, Strauss JD, Heath SG, Zhao KD, Sahota S, et al. The Hand That Gives the Rose. *Mayo ClinProc* 2011; 86(2): 139–144.

## APPENDIX 1: History of Medicine

1. C Keith Wilbur. *Revolutionary Medicine* (Illustrated Living History Series). Globe Pequot Press.
2. Caroline Rance. *History of Medicine in 100 facts*. Amberley Publishing.
3. Helaine Selin. *Medicine Across Cultures: History and Practice of Medicine in Non-Western Cultures* (Science Across Cultures: The History of Non-Western Science). Kluwer Academic Publishers.
4. Henry Ernst Sigerist. *A History of Medicine: I. Primitive and Archaic Medicine*. Oxford University Press Inc Publishers.
5. Henry Ernst Sigerist. *A History of Medicine: II. Early Greek, Hindu, and Persian Medicine*. Oxford University Press Inc Publishers.
6. Jones WHS. *The Doctor's Oath:*
7. Lawrence I Conrad. *The Western Medical Tradition: 800 BC to AD 1800*. Cambridge University Press.
8. Lindberg. *The Beginnings of Western Science*. University of Chicago Press.
9. Lois N Magner. *A History of Medicine*. Taylor and Francis Group Publishers.
10. Osler William. *A Concise History of Medicine* (1919). Kesinger Publication.
11. Paul Strathern. *A Brief History of Medicine: From Hippocrates to Gene Therapy* (Brief Histories). Robinson Publisher.
12. Peter E Pormann. *Medieval Islamic Medicine* (The New Edinburgh Islamic Surveys). Edinburgh University Press.
13. RK Marya. *History of Medicine*. Jaypee Brothers Medical Publishers.
14. Robley Dunglison. *History of Medicine from the Earliest Ages to the Commencement of the Nineteenth Century*. Nabu Press.
15. Roy Porter. *Disease, Medicine and Society in England, 1550–1860* (New Studies in Economic and Social History). Cambridge University Press.

16. Roy Porter. *Greatest Benefit To Mankind: A Medical History of Humanity* (The Norton History of Science). WW Norton Publisher.

17. Roy Porter. *The Cambridge History of Medicine.* Cambridge University Press.

18. Siraisi. *Medieval and Early Renaissance Medicine.* University of Chicago Press.

19. Vivian Nutton. *Ancient Medicine* (Sciences of Antiquity). Routledge publisher.

20. WF Bynum. *Science and the Practice of Medicine in the Nineteenth Century* (Cambridge Studies in the History of Science). Cambridge University Press.

## APPENDIX 2: Hippocratic Oath

1. Kao AC Parsi, KP (September 2004). "Content analyses of oaths administered at U.S. medical schools in 2000". *Academic Medicine* 79 (9): 882–7.

2. Louis Lasagna. *Hippocratic Oath: Modern Version.* Academic Dean of the School of Medicine at Tufts University).

3. Ludwig Edelstein. *The Hippocratic Oath: Text, Translation, and Interpretation.* Baltimore: Johns Hopkins Press, 1943.

4. Sritharan Kaji, Georgina Russell, Zoe Fritz, Davina Wong, Matthew Rollin, Jake Dunning, Bruce Wayne, Philip Morgan, Catherine Sheehan (December 2000). "Medical oaths and declarations". *BMJ* 2001 Dec 22; 323(7327): 1440–1441.

5. von Staden, H (1996). "In a pure and holy way. Personal and professional conduct in the Hippocratic Oath". *Journal of the History of Medicine and Allied Sciences.* 51 (51): 404–437.

6. Wear, Geyer-Kordesch, French (eds) (1993). *Doctors and Ethics: The Earlier Historical Setting of Professional Ethics.* Amsterdam: Rodopi. pp. 10–37.

# Reader's Note

# Reader's Note

# Reader's Note

# Reader's Note